KEY ISSUES IN EVOLVING DEMENTIA CARE

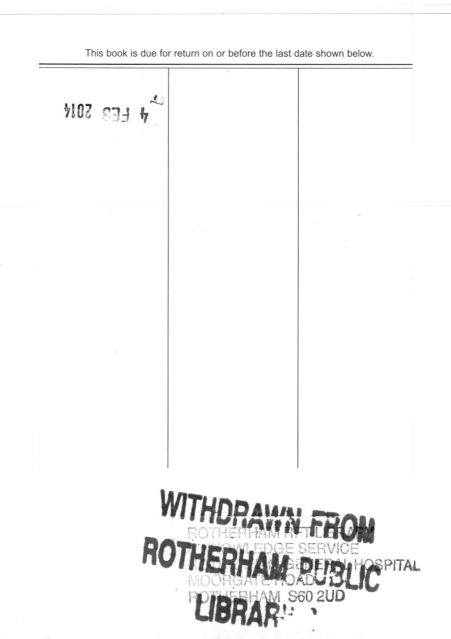

of related interest

Evaluation in Dementia Care
Edited by Anthea Innes and Louise McCabe
ISBN 978 1 84905 242 9
eISBN 978 0 85700 503 8

Dementia and Social Inclusion
Marginalised Groups and Marginalised Areas of
Dementia Research, Care and Practice
Edited by Anthea Innes, Carole Archibald and Charlie Murphy
ISBN 978 1 84310 174 1
eISBN 978 1 84642 025 2

Healing Arts Therapies and Person-Centred Dementia Care
Edited by Anthea Innes and Karen Hatfield
ISBN 978 1 84310 038 6
eISBN 978 1 84642 302 4

Key Issues in Evolving Dementia Care

International Theory-based Policy and Practice

Edited by Anthea Innes, Fiona Kelly
and Louise McCabe

Foreword by Professor June Andrews

Jessica Kingsley *Publishers*
London and Philadelphia

21537

WM 224 INN

First published in 2012
by Jessica Kingsley Publishers
116 Pentonville Road
London N1 9JB, UK
and
400 Market Street, Suite 400
Philadelphia, PA 19106, USA

www.jkp.com

Library of Congress Cataloging in Publication Data
Key issues in evolving dementia care : international theory-based policy and practice / edited by Anthea Innes, Fiona Kelly, and Louise McCabe ; foreword by June Andrews.
    p. cm.
  Includes bibliographical references and index.
  ISBN 978-1-84905-242-9 (alk. paper)
  1. Dementia--Patients--Care--Cross-cultural studies. 2. Dementia--Patients--Care--Government policy.
I. Innes, Anthea. II. Kelly, Fiona, Dr. III. McCabe, Louise.
  RC521.K49 2012
  616.8'3--dc23
                                2011039615

British Library Cataloguing in Publication Data
A CIP catalogue record for this book is available from the British Library

ISBN 978 1 84905 242 9
eISBN 978 0 85700 503 8

Printed and bound in Great Britain

Contents

PART III INNOVATIVE APPROACHES TO CARE

List of Figures, Tables, Boxes and Case studies

FIGURES

Tables

Boxes

Case studies

Foreword

Professor June Andrews

In 2010 the Dementia Services Development Centre at the University of Stirling celebrated its twenty-first birthday. Ironically, at the time we were arranging the party, no one could quite remember or decide when it really started. Was it when the professionals came together in the 1970s, shocked into realisation that there was very little information for professionals about dementia care, and virtually no information for families? Those of us who trained as nurses in the early 1980s could remember being told that dementia was 'a wasting disease' because people with dementia seemed to lose weight and die. We were told not to worry what sort of dementia the person had because it was 'all the same care'. And that was right in a way, because it was a description of what we made happen by the way we worked.

By 1990 Professor Mary Marshall was in Stirling, founding the first centre for developing dementia services in the world. By the turn of the century the Dementia Services Development Trust had raised the funds for the construction of the Iris Murdoch Building in Stirling – the first ever public building built on dementia-friendly principles, and the spiritual home of a worldwide movement to help social care and health care staff working in dementia care to improve services for people with dementia and their families.

The policy interest in dementia in the twenty-first century is largely driven by the realisation that dementia care costs more than cancer, heart disease and stroke put together, in the UK and in other developed countries. Even with this massive spend the media are never short of shocking stories about poor care and people who are so fearful of dementia that they sometimes consider euthanasia as an appropriate response to diagnosis.

So this book is a welcome postscript to our birthday conference. Over 1000 people came to London in October 2010 to celebrate with us. They came from Europe, including the former Soviet Union, the Americas, the Antipodes and Asia, the Far East and Africa – all over the world. Over three days we were inspired by researchers and teachers, inventors and investors, academics and practitioners, and most of all, people with dementia. They inspire us every day.

The papers in this book offer a small selection of the excellent ideas that were presented. After all these years, dementia has truly come of age, and we can use the current policy interest and increased awareness to continue to make change happen on the basis of real evidence and information about what actually makes a difference.

No one wants to have dementia, but until it is eradicated we will continue to work to make things better for those affected. In the beginning, when dementia improvement was in its infancy, anything we did to make it better was good. Now we have come of age, we need to work even harder to continue to make change happen.

Professor June Andrews
Director, Dementia Services Development Centre,
University of Stirling, Scotland

Acknowledgements

The idea for this book stemmed from a conference hosted by the Dementia Services Development Centre in October 2010. Many of the contributors in this collection presented at the conference, and we are delighted that they agreed to develop their presentations into book chapters. Other contributors joined the collection as we developed the idea for the book and identified areas not covered in the conference but that were essential to include in the book.

We would also like to thank Jennifer Anderson for her secretarial assistance when collating the chapters into a full manuscript; her patience and eye for detail were much appreciated.

Introduction

Louise McCabe, Fiona Kelly and Anthea Innes

This book brings together a collection of papers from clinicians, policy influencers and researchers from a range of countries. The book presents theoretical, practice and policy issues demonstrating these three key areas of work in the dementia studies field. Examples from the UK, Malta, India, France, Australia, Canada and the USA are included, providing examples of a range of disciplinary and country-specific initiatives.

The number of people with dementia and people who care for a person with dementia is on the increase. Worldwide the number of people with dementia is estimated to be 35.6 million, with significant predicted increases in coming years (Alzheimer's Disease International 2010). Dementia and the challenges it brings are not limited to western, high-income countries. Currently more than two-thirds of people with dementia live in low- and middle-income countries and these areas are set to see larger increases in the numbers of people with dementia (Ferri *et al.* 2005). The cost of dementia care is also high and predicted to rise due to increasing prevalence and decreased availability of family carers. Currently in the UK dementia care costs more than stroke, heart disease and cancer put together (National Audit Office 2007) and the global cost of dementia in 2010 was estimated at 604 billion US dollars (Alzheimer's Disease International 2010). The balance between the costs associated with informal care, formal social care and medical care differs between regions, although direct medical costs are low in all places. The costs of providing formal social care are high in high-income countries but minimal in low- and middle-income countries where families provide most of the care (Alzheimer's Disease International 2010).

These dramatic figures, alongside developments in understanding dementia and in the provision of support, care and treatment, have led to dementia attracting increased political attention globally. Many countries have developed national plans and strategies and dementia was formally declared a priority by the European Union in 2011 following several years of high-profile campaigning by the French and Belgium presidencies of the European Union. Alzheimer's Disease International continue to campaign for the World Health Organization to similarly prioritise dementia.

This book provides an exploration of theoretical, policy and practice issues that are increasingly important to address, given the projected demographics of dementia care in the future. It also reflects the multidisciplinary nature of dementia studies and the array of academics, practitioners and professionals involved in research and in delivering support, care and treatment to people with dementia and their carers. The contributors represent a range of professions and are drawn from countries that have already identified dementia as a priority area – for example, Australia, England, Scotland, India, France and Malta – as well as countries that are still lobbying for dementia to be recognised as a national priority – for example, Canada and the USA. In this complex field it can be challenging to make the connections between theory, policy and practice. This book will highlight and encourage readers to make these connections and demonstrate that a knowledge of the relationship between theory, policy and practice is required if we are to move discourse around dementia care into the twenty-first century.

The book begins with a theoretical section providing discussion on broader issues relating to dementia and dementia care. The chapters in Part I raise key ideas and issues that underpin policy and practice for people with dementia. In Chapter 1 Innes encourages broad-ranging and interdisciplinary thinking when considering what we mean by dementia and explores the practical impact of differing theoretical perspectives. In order to develop effective policy and practice there is a need to understand the real impact of dementia in both social and economic terms, and Chapter 2 by Dudgeon addresses these questions through a case study from Canada. In Chapter 3 Coley, Berr and Andrieu review current evidence on prevalence and risk factors for dementia, demonstrating avenues for future policy and practice. Finally, in Chapter 4, Telford, Gallagher and Reynish present a discussion on how services can work innovatively to meet the changing needs of older people with dementia, examining the influence of theory on practice. The chapters in Part I give readers of the book 'hooks' to understand the later chapters and also to consider their own practice context.

Part II focuses on national dementia strategies and plans. Around the world, countries are developing policy for the treatment and care of people with dementia in a strategic manner, often in the form of a national strategy or plan. A series of case studies is presented from England, France, Scotland and Malta. The national strategy in England (Chapter 5) is highly regarded and has achieved clear recognition from government in the UK. France was one of the first countries to develop a national plan with full support from their government (Chapter 6). The work in France is of particular importance as it helped to promote Europe-wide recognition of dementia care, supported by the French presidency of the European Union in 2007–2008. A regional strategy from Scotland is presented in Chapter 7, providing evidence for the importance of local policy development. The Malta case study in Chapter 8 demonstrates that even in a small country with relatively few resources it is still possible to develop a strategic approach to improving dementia care.

Part III of the book integrates policy and theory with four practice chapters spanning the UK, India, Australia and the USA, and examines key and topical dementia care practice issues within these regions. In Chapter 9 some of the difficulties and barriers encountered by people newly diagnosed with dementia and their family members when accessing post-diagnostic support and services in the UK are compared and explored, and holistic ways in which services can meet the needs of people with dementia in the UK and beyond are presented. A programme delivering education and support to family carers in Goa, India, is presented in Chapter 10, demonstrating innovative approaches to improving the lives of people with dementia in a low-income country. Chapter 11 reports on a study from Australia evaluating the impact of the environment on physical activity levels of people with dementia in residential care settings. Chapter 12 reports on an innovative way to engage and educate staff and families of people with dementia in long-term care in Louisiana, USA – one of the most impoverished and racially divided regions of the country.

The book concludes by drawing together the key issues raised within the chapters to demonstrate and illustrate links between theory, policy and practice, as well as identifying gaps that need to be addressed to ensure that dementia is approached holistically, in a way that addresses theory–practice and policy–practice gaps. In this way future directions are suggested that take account of dementia-specific policy, early detection and diagnosis of dementia, conceptualisations of dementia, the views of people with dementia and an agenda of innovation and change.

Theory and dementia

Since the late 1980s there has been a rise in the number of practitioners and academics who are concerned with conceptualisations of dementia. In a remarkably short period of time we have seen biomedical constructs of dementia challenged (Bond 1992; Lyman 1989), a focus on the experiences of the individual with dementia (Kitwood 1997) and a realisation and acknowledgement that those with dementia have insight and awareness into their condition (Clare 2004). There has been a growing engagement from social science and social gerontology, bringing an appreciation of the social structures that shape the experience of dementia and the way care practices are defined and carried out (Innes 2009). No longer is it acceptable to understand dementia as a disease constructed within negative images of decline and degeneration to the point of death. The active lobbying of people with dementia to bring about political and practice changes and to improve understanding of dementia exemplifies the importance of a move away from the traditional control of dementia by professionals to a real engagement with those who can tell us most about what dementia involves: those with the diagnosis. Examples of the inspiring impact made by those with dementia on understandings of dementia are found in our own country (Scotland) and internationally. Members of the Scottish Dementia Working Group[1] are in demand to present at international events and have been active participants in the development of the Scottish Dementia Strategy. Worldwide the Dementia Advocacy and Support Network International (DASNI)[2] has seen people with dementia from across the globe come together and share their experiences and ideas; members of this network have written and talked about dementia and provide a clear message – that people with dementia cannot be overlooked when talking about what dementia is and what it means to live with it. Therefore theorising about dementia is not an ivory tower activity, but one that demands an understanding of complex disciplinary and professional perspectives and to ensure that the voice of those with dementia is at the centre of discourse.

In the dementia studies field, 'theory' refers to the different starting points, perspectives and approaches that those working in the field as practitioners, policy makers, researchers and carers, and those with dementia, use to describe and understand dementia, and in turn how they then operationalise these ideas in their delivery of care, development of policy, or understanding of their lived experiences. Innes begins Part I of this book by outlining three influential theoretical perspectives for understanding dementia, namely biomedical, psychological and gerontological. She argues for a need to appreciate the strengths of each perspective and to understand the impact that different theoretical starting points have for how policy is developed, the practices that will be advocated on the ground and the type of research that will be conducted. In this way a holistic approach to understanding dementia may evolve, one that uses the strengths of different perspectives to provide the best possible care for people with dementia and support for their carers (paid and unpaid), and to influence policy that will support high-quality care practices.

Dudgeon (Chapter 2) provides an interesting example of how to approach policy by influencing understanding of the key issues that will impact on the

---

1   For more information on this organisation see www.sdwg.org.uk.
2   For more information on this organisation see www.dasninternational.org.

cost of providing high-quality dementia care to those with dementia, and appropriate support for carers and professionals. Dudgeon outlines a complex process used to develop a compelling document presented to policy makers to bring about desired policy and practice changes. This chapter is very much an exemplar of using understandings of dementia to bring about lasting change supported at the highest level of government.

Coley, Berr and Andrieu (Chapter 3) provide an overview of epidemiological research and the risk factors that might be modifiable, such as lifestyle factors (smoking, alcohol, exercise and diet) and vascular factors (such as diabetes and high blood pressure) that could be prevented by modifying lifestyle factors. However, they conclude that interventions focused on these factors have so far been unsuccessful when tested in research. Therefore medical practices for treating dementia or for trying to prevent dementia are based on limited scientific research. They do, however, highlight that factors associated with healthy living generally will not be harmful, and could be beneficial in reducing the risk of developing dementia in the future.

Telford, Gallagher and Reynish (Chapter 4) provide an example of putting into practice ideas for treatment, management and care for people with dementia. They discuss the importance of diagnosis, prevalence and different forms of dementia, for the management and treatment plans that are put into practice for those with dementia. They argue for a multicomponent approach that takes account of a multitude of factors to work towards delivering holistic care.

Policy and dementia

Policy is crucial, as it influences how care and treatment are delivered to people with dementia and the outcomes experienced by them and their carers. Policy is in turn influenced by research and theoretical developments in the field of dementia studies; hence the placement of the policy chapters in the middle of this book.

Historically, people with dementia have not been considered as a priority group within policy in the UK and other countries. Cook (2008) reviewed policy in Scotland and England and found that until 2007 there had been little mention of dementia in policy. The *National Service Framework for Older People* was one of the few policy documents published in the UK that discussed the needs of people with dementia and recommended specialist services for them (Department of Health 2001). Recently, however, it would appear that activity in the field of dementia care and treatment has reached a point where there is a recognised need at governmental levels for specific policy to address the needs of people with dementia and their carers. There also seems to be political will in many countries to address these issues. This increasing awareness and willingness to act are no doubt linked to the predicted dramatic rise in numbers of people with dementia, but also to changes in our understanding of dementia care and the needs of people with dementia and their carers, highlighted in many chapters in this book.

Responses to these changes are evidenced in the growing number of regional and national dementia strategies and plans being developed, or already published, in countries across Europe and other parts of the world. These seek to improve care and support for people with dementia by providing clear frameworks for the delivery of treatment and services for people with dementia and their carers. Dementia strategies are particularly interesting when considering the overall approach to dementia care and support in an individual country, region or culture. They may not be tied to one discipline or sector, and so can give a picture of the general policy approach to dementia care in that country and the key pieces of legislation that frame delivery of care and treatment. Strategies are also aspirational, and therefore reflect current thinking about dementia care in that region. To date England, France, Norway and Scotland, among others, have launched national dementia plans and strategies, with many more in the process of developing such strategies.[3] Other countries have developed approaches to improving the experiences of people with dementia and their carers, although these have not been published as discrete plans. For example, Korea has declared 'war on dementia' (Lee 2010, p.931) and Japan's Ministry of Health, Labour and Welfare is promoting a range of strategies 'to establish an appropriate support system for people with dementia' (Arai, Arai and Mizuno 2010, p.896).

Many of the strategies have similar aims, specifically: to improve public awareness of dementia; to improve diagnostic processes and increase rates of earlier diagnosis; and to improve the quality of current care services. Most also mention the importance of research. Many of the national strategies do not have funding attached, and improvements in services have to take place by diverting funds from elsewhere. This makes implementation of such strategies particularly challenging.

Part II of this book presents four chapters focusing on processes of development, implementation and outcomes of dementia strategies from different countries and regions. Three national strategies (from England, Malta and France) are presented, along with one regional strategy from Fife in Scotland. In Chapter 5 Banerjee provides a detailed account of the background context and development process for the English national

---

3   Up-to-date information on national dementia strategies across Europe can be found on the Alzheimer Europe website. See www.alzheimer-europe.org/EN/Policy-in-Practice2/National-Dementia-Plans.

dementia strategy that was published in 2009, as well as commenting on the success of implementation to date. In his discussion of implementation Banerjee illustrates many of the challenges and barriers faced at the national level. A series of Alzheimer plans have been published in France since 2001 and Guisset-Martinez (Chapter 6) provides background information on these plans, focusing on the most recent plan published in 2008. Key areas of successful development in health and social care for people with dementia and their carers in France are highlighted. Chapter 7 presents a case study of a regional strategy from Fife, an area in East Scotland. McCabe describes the processes undertaken to develop the strategy and provides examples of projects that have been influenced by the strategy, highlighting good practice that has resulted from the strategy development project and demonstrating the importance of local policy and planning. This is followed by Scerri's (Chapter 8) presentation of results from a survey undertaken in Malta to gather information on dementia care and views on how a dementia strategy might be designed and implemented. This early stage in strategy development highlights the importance of involving a broad range of stakeholders and illustrates the usefulness of collecting diverse data, both to support and to guide strategy development. Each chapter in Part II adds to our understanding of dementia strategies and how these develop and influence care and treatment for people with dementia in different areas. The chapters also provide insights into the policy and planning processes and how these influence country-specific political and cultural contexts.

Dementia practice

One of the many *Oxford English Dictionary* definitions of practice is: 'action or execution as opposed to theory'. For those working in health, allied health and social services this means working to implement policy, meet goals and targets, advance learning and reflect on practice in order to deliver better care and support. However, 'practice' is not a unified concept. As we will see in Part III, for different professions it means different philosophies of working, and for different cultures it is influenced by different understandings of dementia (Innes 2009), often with implications for those in receipt of such practices. In relation to 'care', a term with mixed appeal, particularly for those providing informal or unpaid care to a person with dementia (Carpenter and Mak 2007), care of people with dementia, particularly as their condition progresses, is usually formalised and provided by paid workers in Western Europe and North America – although in low- and middle-income countries family members are still the main source of care and support. Glendinning *et al.* (2009) found that, throughout the European Union, patterns of informal care, society's attitudes towards family responsibilities, and the availability of services to support older and disabled people and/or carers all vary widely between member states. These differences are reflected in the lower quality of life reported by carers in Mediterranean and Eastern European countries, compared to countries with developed welfare services like the UK and Sweden.

In the UK the policy drive towards self-directed care under the ethos of personalisation has entered the dementia practice agenda (Simmons 2009) and is beginning to influence how care is delivered by practitioners and experienced by people with dementia and their families. Further, as policy has moved forward in recognising that people with dementia, their families and those who support them have specific, often unmet, needs, practitioners and others have also recognised unmet needs and sought ways to address these, often through innovative means. Part III of this book focuses on three key areas identified as crucial to the experiences of people with dementia and their families and essential for those who support and care for them: the necessity for staff training, the importance of an early diagnosis and ongoing post-diagnostic support, and the value for well-being of dementia-friendly environments. The contributors to the four chapters in Part III take an applied approach and illustrate, from the perspectives of those providing support and those receiving support, the barriers, opportunities and consequences of policy and specific contexts of care that have a bearing on those within the care environment. In Chapter 9 Kelly and Szymczynska examine the evolution of memory services in urban and rural regions of Scotland in response to government policy; specifically the functioning of memory clinics and the provision of post-diagnostic support to people newly diagnosed with dementia and their families. Areas of interest include the role of community services, education and training needs of families, and challenges experienced by professionals. In a rapidly changing economic climate, ensuring that policy is carried out in practice requires scrutiny of difficulties (whether organisational, practical or personal), and Chapter 9 highlights some of the areas where good practice might be hampered, despite the best of intentions of those working to provide a good service.

Dias (Chapter 10) presents the changing culture and contexts of caring for people with dementia in India – a country that is home to one sixth of the world's population and which is undergoing huge demographic and cultural change, resulting in changes to family care practices and experiences. Dias presents findings from an evaluation of an innovative project using community-based care workers to support family members to cope with difficulties in caring for family members with dementia at home. This is an excellent example of the value in using local resources, in this case people with local knowledge, to achieve a positive outcome for family carers and ultimately for people with dementia living at home.

In Chapter 11 deVries and Traynor report on a study examining the relationship between physical design of a care setting in Australia and the physical activity levels of people with dementia who lived there. Their findings point to the lack of consideration given in practice to ensuring that the built environment facilitates walking for people with dementia, beyond that which occurs as part of daily routine. This is despite the plethora of literature promoting activity as being conducive to well-being of people with dementia (Weuve *et al.* 2004; Zeisel 2006). deVries and Traynor usefully integrate their empirical findings with the research literature to present recommendations to practitioners, managers, educators and care providers for modifying the design of care environments to promote increased activity levels of those who live there.

Finally, in Chapter 12 Johnson and Johnson move the focus from practice to supporting education and training of paid caregivers in the Southern regions of America. They describe the challenges they encountered while delivering dementia education and training to black certified nursing aides (CNAs), recognised as a marginalised group of workers. Their contextualising descriptions of the difficulties experienced by these workers (racism, domestic stress and discrimination) offer important insight into how the cultural context impacts on the world of work and influences workers' experiences of carrying out care for people with dementia.

All four chapters in Part III take an applied approach and report on innovative ways in which issues identified in policy, or arising as a result of policy, have been addressed. Befitting an applied approach and an interest in the experiences of people, some contributors (Dias; deVries and Traynor) have used case studies, while others (Kelly and Szymczynska; Johnson and Johnson) have used direct quotes from participants to illustrate key findings from their studies. In these ways, we hear in the words of those experiencing care and support, and those delivering care and support, the issues of importance to them and the consequences for them of changing demographics, economics, policies or circumstances.

Summary

Dementia is one of the key health challenges of the twenty-first century. Demographic predictions show huge increases in the numbers of people affected by the condition, as well as changing patterns in the delivery of care and support available for people with dementia. To address these challenges and to enable good quality and appropriate care to be provided for everyone with dementia, policy makers, professionals and practitioners in the dementia field need to develop ever more innovative approaches to dementia policy and service provision. The chapters in this book provide some examples of innovative policy and innovative approaches to working with people with dementia and those who care for and support them. Identifying challenges and barriers to change is a fundamental step towards instituting change, and this book offers examples in policy and practice where some of these challenges have been addressed.

References

Alzheimer's Disease International (ADI) (2010) *The World Alzheimer's Report*. London: ADI.

Arai, Y., Arai, A. and Mizuno, Y. (2010) 'The national dementia strategy in Japan.' *International Journal of Geriatric Psychiatry 25*, 896–899.

Bond, J. (1992) 'The medicalization of dementia.' *Journal of Aging Studies 6*, 4, 397–403.

Carpenter, B. and Mak, W. (2007) 'Caregiving couples.' *Generations*, Fall Issue, 47–53.

Clare, L. (2004) 'Awareness in early-stage Alzheimer's disease: a review of methods and evidence.' *British Journal of Clinical Psychology 43*, 2, 177–196.

Cook, A. (2008) *Dementia and Well Being* (Policy and Practice in Health and Social Care Series). Edinburgh: Dunedin Academic Press.

Department of Health (2001) *National Service Framework for Older People*. London: Department of Health.

Ferri, C., Prince, M., Brayne, C., Brodaty, H. *et al.* for Alzheimer's Disease International (2005) 'Global prevalence of dementia: a Delphi consensus study.' *The Lancet 366*, 2112–2117.

Glendinning, C., Arksey, H., Tjadens, F., Morée, M., Moran, N. and Nies, H. (2009) *Care Provision within Families and its Socio-Economic Impact on Care Providers across the European Union*. York: University of York, Social Policy Research Unit.

Innes, A. (2009) *Dementia Studies: A Social Science Perspective*. London: Sage.

Kitwood, T. (1997) *Dementia Reconsidered: The Person Comes First*. Buckingham: Open University Press.

Lee, S. (2010) 'Dementia strategy Korea.' *International Journal of Geriatric Psychiatry 25*, 931–932.

Lyman, K.A. (1989) 'Bringing the social back in: a critique of the bio-medicalisation of dementia.' *The Gerontologist 29*, 5, 597–604.

National Audit Office (2007) *Improving Services and Support for People with Dementia*. London: National Audit Office.

Simmons, H. (2009) 'Personalising dementia care in Scotland.' *Journal of Care Services Management 4*, 1, 10–15.

Weuve, J., Kang, J.H., Manson, J.E., Breteler, M.B., Ware, J.H. and Grodstein, F. (2004) 'Physical activity, including walking, and cognitive function in older women.' *Journal of the American Medical Association 292*, 12, 1454–1461.

Zeisel, J. (2006) *Inquiry by Design*. New York: WW Norton and Co.

Part I

CONCEPTUALISING DEMENTIA

Chapter 1

Towards a Holistic Approach for Understanding Dementia

Anthea Innes

Summary

Dementia attracts a multidisciplinary and multiprofessional audience and therefore a wide array of ideas and conceptualisations about dementia. This chapter discusses three different theoretical approaches that contribute to our understanding of dementia. These can be broadly distinguished as biomedical, psychosocial and gerontological perspectives, and all have made theoretical contributions to the dementia field. These three broad theoretical models underpin aspects of dementia care policy, practice and research. This chapter begins by providing an overview of each of the three approaches: biomedical, psychosocial and critical social-gerontological. The contribution and implications of each theoretical model that shape our understandings of dementia will then be discussed. The chapter concludes by providing examples of how a more holistic approach to theoretical understandings of dementia could be used to shape and inform policy, practice and research. It is imperative to understand the different starting points of different professions and disciplines that are involved in the study of dementia and provide dementia care services, if the goal is to achieve an integrated model of dementia that encompasses theory, policy and practice.

Introduction

Dementia is a condition attracting increasing global attention and policy concern. Demographic changes have led to projections of an increase in the number of people with dementia at a time when there are fewer people of working age available to provide care. There are an estimated 35.6 million people with dementia worldwide and it is projected that by 2050 this figure will have increased to over 115 million (Alzheimer's Disease International 2010). Building on the robust calculations from Knapp *et al.* (2007), the

Alzheimer Society estimate there to be 634,030 with dementia in England alone (Alzheimer Society 2011). Dementia is now a national priority in many countries worldwide, with Australia being the first country to adopt a dementia strategy. Other countries have followed this example. In the UK there are dementia strategies for England (Department of Health 2009) and Scotland (Scottish Government 2010), and a consultation process in Northern Ireland for a regional dementia strategy (DHSSPS 2010) conducted in 2010 (Innes *et al.* 2010) was made available on the DHSSPS website in 2011.

The UK provides a clear indication of government recognition of the 'demographic time bomb' (Knapp *et al.* 2007) or 'epidemic' (Wilson and Fearnley 2007) that dementia represents. This concern is reflected at a pan-European level. The 2007–2008 French presidency of the European Union pledged support for dementia to be a European priority. Growing pressure, driven by France, for dementia to be made a European priority (Alzheimer Europe 2008) led to a written declaration on Alzheimer's disease by the European Parliament in 2011 (European Parliament 2011).

Governments and consumer groups worldwide are concerned with how to best provide care for people with dementia. This concern is in part influenced by the cost of dementia care. In the UK, dementia currently incurs a yearly cost of £17bn (Knapp *et al.* 2007), costing the nation more than cancer, stroke and heart disease put together (National Audit Office 2007). Dementia is set to become one of the key health challenges of the twenty-first century. Yet how best to provide care and support to people with dementia and their carers within fiscal constraints remains a challenge. This is in part due to a lack of theoretical development in the field that would clearly conceptualise dementia and what this means for high quality care delivery and the policy drivers that shape care practices.

For over 100 years there has been interest in dementia from biomedical disciplines and health professions, where the key concern was around understanding the disease process (Dillman 2000; Holstein 1997). A more recent disciplinary interest in dementia emerged from social psychology in the 1980s, and the result is a key concern with examining how the disease might impact on the individual who has dementia (Kitwood 1997; Sabat 2001). Social gerontology, in particular critical social gerontology, has been important in raising critiques of biomedical approaches to dementia (Bond 1992; Lyman 1989), highlighting the need to consider the wider social context of dementia care (Innes 2002).

Theory refers to the ideas, conceptualisations, perspectives and approaches that different academic disciplines, professions and lay people may hold about dementia. However, what is less well understood are the theoretical starting points that influence policy and shape what is considered to be good practice.

Because dementia attracts multidisciplinary and multiprofessional interest, the discourse around dementia care practice is such that the underlying assumptions of recommendations are blurred or implicit. Therefore an integrated understanding of the theoretical approaches that underpin the dementia studies field is required. To do this means that it is vital not only to understand one particular perspective when approaching the study of dementia and how this shapes policy, practice and research directives, but also to be aware of the multiple theories that shape dementia discourse.

This chapter begins by critically assessing three influential theoretical approaches to understanding and conceptualising dementia. It then moves on to discuss examples of how each theoretical approach contributes to knowledge and understanding of dementia, which in turn shapes new theory and knowledge generation. It is proposed that an integrated model for approaching the study of dementia is needed to advance future dementia policy and practice.

Different theoretical approaches

Dementia attracts the attention of an interdisciplinary audience in terms of professional backgrounds, for example nursing, social work, medicine and other allied health professions. It also attracts multiple academic disciplines as diverse as sociology and pharmacology. Therefore what we know about dementia, or what we think we know about dementia, comes from diverse sources, diverse starting points and diverse interests. Different theoretical models, perspectives or approaches are often used in a commonplace way when discussing dementia. This has resulted in a situation where we can have 'confused professionals' (Harding and Palfrey 1997), who do not necessarily understand what dementia is, nor the best way to approach the care of those diagnosed. If we wish to study dementia, learn more about this condition and improve the services and support we offer to those with dementia, it is critical for us to have an understanding and critical appreciation of the contribution different approaches offer to our knowledge and practice base, and of how this in turn shapes and is shaped by policy and research.

Biomedical perspectives

History demonstrates that people with dementia were viewed as vulnerable and cast as different (Dillman 2000). When this happens a process of stigmatisation can occur (Goffman 1963). Research on stigma and dementia is limited (Poveda 2003) but was acknowledged in a Scottish study with the mainstream population (Devlin, MacAskill and Stead 2007), demonstrating that such a view remains within society today.

The biomedical model has three main propositions:

- Dementia is a pathological, abnormal condition.

- Dementia is organic in aetiology and progresses through stages.

- Dementia is diagnosed using biomedical assessments.

(Lyman 1989)

To view dementia as pathological it is necessary to define what is normal, but it may be difficult to distinguish between dementia and normal aging (Gubrium 1986). Although those providing dementia care may have altered their practices over time and it is now widely recognised that dementia refers to a set of symptoms rather than a disease in and of itself, the theoretical foundations of biomedical perspectives remain. There is a fine boundary between what is accepted as normal behaviour and that attributed to a biomedical or psychological condition, as has been demonstrated in discussions of mental illness (Crisp *et al.* 2000). It has also been found that behaviours that an individual has displayed throughout their lifetime may, following diagnosis, be attributed to the effects of dementia (Lyman 1989). The label of dementia also changes the way people interact with someone with dementia (Harding and Palfrey 1997).

The supposedly stage-like progression of dementia that is used in biomedical discourses of dementia has been criticised. This is because progression of symptoms is highly variable and distinct stages are rarely seen (Gubrium 1986). Carers, however, often accept the existence of stages, as this offers some explanation for the behaviour of the individual with dementia and a degree of prediction about future events (Kitwood 1997). A tension for the carer may, however, develop when the disease progression does not fit with the given stage (Gubrium 1986).

Medical treatment of dementia leads to a power relationship between doctors and carers and the person with dementia. When a carer is under stress they may exert more control on the individual with dementia, and this may be done, within the biomedical model, using chemical restraints (Lyman 1989). This power relationship may have a detrimental effect on the behaviour of the person with dementia (Bond 1992; Lyman 1989). It may also have a negative outcome in that the carer may start to expect deterioration in the individual's condition and behaviour. Dementia could thus become a self-fulfilling prophecy (Lyman 1989).

Biomedical perspectives on dementia make a useful contribution to caring (Bond 1992), as the conception of dementia as a medical problem provides a way of coping with the challenges of caring for a person with dementia. It also offers an explanation for what is happening to the person with dementia (Bond 1992). In addition both carers and doctors benefit from a disease label for dementia (Harding and Palfrey 1997). Biomedical perspectives are also useful in that they provide a differential diagnosis, and treatment for other conditions which can exacerbate symptoms of dementia (e.g. infection or hypothyroidism). There are therefore important aspects to biomedical models of dementia that can help nurses to negotiate their role with other professionals and with carers. Labelling dementia as a disease can also help to reduce the stigma often associated with conditions seen as mental health problems, and it has been argued that the medicalisation of dementia led to increased research funding for Alzheimer's disease and other types of dementia (Fox 2000). Biomedical approaches have done much to alert us to the importance of early diagnosis and possible ways to protect against developing dementia in later life. The primary element that is missing from biomedical accounts of dementia is the views and experiences of the person with dementia. Biomedical models have been argued to have limitations in their usefulness, as illustrated by Harding and Palfrey (1997, p.34) when they summarise what is known about dementia from empirically based research: 'cause: unknown; diagnosis: very difficult until after death'. However, this argument is weakening, given the advances in diagnostic procedures such as magnetic resonance imaging, the growth in the prescribing of anti-dementia drugs, and increased awareness of factors that may prevent or pose a risk for developing dementia in later life. The key remaining gap in biomedical accounts of dementia is the omission of the viewpoint of the individual with dementia.

Social-psychological perspectives

Critiques of biomedical approaches have paved the way for alternative conceptualisations of dementia based on social-psychological perspectives. On both sides of the Atlantic at around the same time, during the late 1980s and early 1990s, Tom Kitwood (UK) and Steven Sabat (US) both independently began advancing alternative understandings to the decline, decay and deficiency models of dementia commonly promoted by those working within an approach defined by biomedical understandings.

Kitwood's work (1990, 1993, 1997) can be considered as a deconstruction of the medical model of dementia, but he did not deny the biomedical basis of dementia. His key contribution to understanding dementia, and in the process challenging the medical model of care, was his insistence that what he termed 'personhood' – defined as 'a status or standing bestowed upon one human being, by others, in the context of social relationship and social being. It implies recognition, respect and trust' (1997, p.8) – should be preserved, even if a person received the diagnosis of dementia. Consequently, maintaining personhood means that we enter into partnership with that person and assist them to maintain an identity and worth through our interactions and communication strategies, and this issue is one that has continuing relevance to care practice (e.g. Cowdell 2006; Dewing 2008; Edvardsson, Winblad and Sandman 2008).

A further contribution to social-psychological discourse on dementia began with Sabat and Harré (1992), who argued for the importance of recognising the self of people with dementia. Sabat (1994, 2001, 2002, 2006) has gone on to develop this line of thinking and has argued that there are three forms of self:

- *Self 1:* this is the singular self and uses the indexicals of 'I, me, mine' to describe personal attributes. For example, 'I like that, those belong to me, those are mine.'

- *Self 2:* this aspect of self consists of the characteristics held by an individual (mental, physical and emotional), and the beliefs the individual holds about these characteristics or attributes. For example, 'I am good at cooking,' or conversely 'I am hopeless at cooking.'

- *Self 3:* this is the publicly presented persona that requires the co-operation of others. For example, in the roles and relationships an individual holds (worker, parent, friend, etc.).

Sabat has used case studies to exemplify the importance of acknowledging the different aspects of self. However, he argues that the most vulnerable or fragile self is Self 3 (Sabat 2006), as this requires skilled caregiving and interactions to uphold previous relationships and roles.

A further, more recent and relevant contribution made by social-psychology to understanding dementia is through work focusing on the concept of awareness (Clare 2003, 2004), where it has been shown that people with dementia do have insight into their condition and that there are a variety of ways to elicit this information. Hughes (2011) suggests a 'human-person perspective' which takes account of the standing a person has in the world in relationship with others. In many ways this approach resonates with the person-centred approach advocated by Kitwood (1997), but it develops thinking regarding what this means about how to act rather than simply to reflect.

However, person-centred care is perhaps the most enduring contribution to the dementia field that began with Kitwood's (1997) application of psychological perspectives to dementia. This is in part because person-centred care provides practitioners with a framework of values that are ethical, humanitarian and respectful of the person with dementia (Edvardsson *et al.* 2008). Kelly (2010) argues that focusing on the selves of people with dementia may offer practitioners a way to provide person-centred care. It is interesting that this parallels Sabat's own work (1994) where he brought together ideas from person-centred care alongside his conceptualisations on the self. Yet there remains an elusive lack of evidence about what aspects of person-centred care work, and what is required to achieve person-centred care (e.g. personal attributes of staff members or organisational structures; Innes, Macpherson and McCabe 2006). Despite the rhetoric of person-centred care and anecdotal accounts of person-centred care in practice, outcome measures for person-centred care remain elusive, as does widespread change in care practices. This is because person-centred care does not focus on the wider social and political context that surrounds care provision and understandings of dementia, nor does it provide a change strategy to deliver high quality care. The concepts of self and awareness place more emphasis on the way the person with dementia continues to express their self-identity and demonstrate awareness of their condition and their environment.

Social psychology has done much to remind carers and professionals of the importance of focusing on the individual person with dementia. It highlights possible therapies and interventions that might be useful for an individual, or for their family to help them support the person with dementia. The importance of finding therapies that suit an individual has been stressed, as has providing early interventions to try and help the individual minimise disabilities associated with developing dementia symptoms over time. Yet the focus on the individual with dementia, while representing an important move forward in the dementia field, does not examine the wider factors that place people with dementia in a position that is often marginal and low status. As such, psychology does not offer answers or suggestions about how to improve the overall place of people with dementia in society. The overall limitation of psychological perspectives is the failure to locate analysis of experiences of individuals within wider social, political, cultural and economic concerns which combine to shape the experiences of individuals and the care that they receive.

Theoretical approaches to understanding dementia stemming from sociology and social gerontology do offer such opportunities.

Critical social gerontology

First and foremost, gerontology looks at the place and status of older people in society. Initially work in the gerontology field focused on political economy, and in particular the burden of older people on society (Walker and Phillipson 1986), and later began, through critical gerontology, to move on and look at the disadvantages faced by older people in society.

Social gerontology alerts us to the discrimination faced by older people in western societies and highlights the cross-cutting interplay of gender, class and age (Dressel, Minkler and Yen 1997) on aging experiences. Given the ageist social context people with dementia are located within, it is perhaps unsurprising to discover that the initial theoretical work pushed towards medicalising this condition and the avoidance of engaging with the lived realities of people with dementia. Critical social gerontology examines taken-for-granted structural inequalities and power dynamics which perpetuate current understandings of aging (Estes, Biggs and Phillipson 2003), and this is important as it raises a challenge to the negative connotations that the label dementia has traditionally held, and continues to hold, within society.

Applying more positive frameworks to the experience of dementia is an important way forward. For example, the notion of successful aging is being applied to the experience of dementia. Harris (2008) argues that the concept of resilience has been overlooked when it comes to dementia, and that such a concept is useful when considering successful aging. She provides case study examples of how people with dementia have remained resilient throughout their dementia and so continue to age successfully while negotiating the label dementia. Harris and Keady (2008) argue that more positive conceptualisations of dementia are needed for images of dementia to alter and for the stigma surrounding dementia to be broken down. This presents a challenge for dementia care, one where success in living with dementia can be identified, progressing from the old biomedical view of dementia as a disease of decline and decay with no hope of cure, to consideration of a life with dementia that can remain fulfilling.

Gerontology initially overlooked privileged groups. However, the presence of multiple privileges as well as multiple oppressions is important for helping us to understand the experiences of different groups of older people and people with dementia in our societies (Hulko 2004). Gerontologists were slow to include gender, class and race differences (amongst others) as a focus of enquiry; now there is a great deal of work looking at gender differences in particular.

In critiquing and deconstructing disease labels there is a danger that the very real medical symptoms of illness could be overlooked. Therefore it is important to remain alert to the contributions of biomedical accounts. The final critique that can be made of gerontology is that dementia was not an immediate area of interest for gerontological researchers. However, gerontology now encompasses much work that is being done in the dementia studies field and plays an important part in reminding us of the wider social and structural factors that shape an individual's experience of dementia, an experience that goes beyond the presence of symptoms diagnosed as dementia.

As the number and proportion of older people and people with dementia increases in industrialised countries, the reputation of dementia as an illness and the stigma associated with it will need to be challenged. If we are sincere in desiring to adopt holistic approaches and empower the person with dementia, then we need to recognise that there is 'life beyond the illness' (Goldsmith 1996); we need to see the person first, before the label of dementia, and we need to resist ageist assumptions that are endemic throughout western societies. Geronotology is therefore an important perspective to consider when thinking about dementia, as it reminds us of wider society and goes beyond both the individualism promoted by social psychology, and the disease labelling of biomedical perspectives. Gerontology reminds us of disadvantage and discrimination experienced by older people, and most recently it has become concerned with promoting the voice of older people. This is a trend mirrored in the dementia care field where there is greater emphasis and concern about hearing the views of service users and their carers (Innes 2009).

How we approach dementia, and what our starting point is, whether professionally and/or academically or as a policy maker, will have an impact on how we see the 'problem'; how we might try to approach it; and how we might try and respond to it or look for a solution. As can be seen from the brief overview and critique above of what are arguably the three overarching theoretical approaches that have generated knowledge about dementia, there are quite different starting points for approaching dementia policy, practice and research.

Figure 1.1 is based on the idea of a web of understanding of dementia that leads to the (re)generation, production and challenge to knowledge that has been put forward and discussed by Innes (2009). This figure, although necessarily simplifying aspects of a complex process for illustrative purposes, shows that the way dementia is conceptualised will have a particular impact on the policy developments that may take place. This in turn will promote a certain kind of care practice that will be subject to research scrutiny, which may reproduce, rather than challenge, thinking, instead of generating new knowledge. Thus, a 'web of understanding' is a useful tool for thinking about how conceptualisation of dementia can impact on the knowledge that is generated about dementia, the policy frameworks that will shape care practice, and the focus that research will adopt.

It is clear that biomedical perspectives have dominated dementia discourse for the last century (Harding and Palfrey 1997), and although this has been subject to a robust critique, biomedical proponents have managed to raise the profile of the condition by focusing on the prevalence and incidence of dementia, which will probably lead to huge increases in the numbers of people who will experience dementia this century (Knapp *et al.* 2007). The importance of early diagnosis and preventative measures means, however, that care services will in future be much more responsive to the needs expressed by people with dementia and their carers. The costs of dementia to society make it possible, in the context of social policy and health and social care systems, to highlight the experience of dementia in a very stark way that grabs political attention. Earlier diagnosis will mean more opportunities for active engagement in society, and perhaps a focus on a successful model of aging, while enabling individualised care and treatment packages to be devised. Across the UK dementia policy has focused on the need to diagnose dementia earlier and to ensure that diagnostic processes are developed to help meet government objectives or targets.

The undoubted contribution of social psychology to dementia discourses lies in its focus on the individual with dementia. Challenging the underlying assumption of the loss of the person, which the disease label has promoted, has offered practitioners the opportunity to focus on providing individualised care to people with dementia. Focusing on the individual has led to the development of models for practice where core values can be applied to nursing (McCormack 2004) and social work practice (Parker 2005). This has been embraced by many practitioners as it offers an alternative to a warehousing model, where the focus is merely on meeting basic human care needs for warmth and nourishment, and reports which demonstrate that universal high standards of individualised care are still lacking (Age Concern England 2007; National Audit Office 2007) are now contributing to the drive behind policy developments.

Therefore, despite the appeal that social psychology may have for practitioners, making this a reality supported by policy is problematic; and this is largely due to the micro-level focus on caring for an individual, which is dependent on the personal skills of individual health and social care professionals.

By contrast, understanding of dementia from a gerontological perspective moves on from a focus on the individual, micro-level of analysis and examines wider structural issues. Understanding dementia from a gerontological viewpoint requires acknowledging the position of older people within society and how the disease label 'dementia' impacts on their lived experiences – experiences that are shaped and structured by wider social forces. Care practices would be fully assessed from the point of view of service users (and other stakeholders), rather than by the often tokenistic approach that is generally used, and the notion of successful aging could become an alternative to negative images of those with dementia when examining users' lives. Research would ensure that the views of people with dementia were collated, and that the findings were placed within the social, political, cultural and economic context in which the person lived.

Working in the dementia field demands an appreciation of the contributions of different theoretical and disciplinary approaches, as the contributions from different perspectives can together help to improve the lives of people with dementia. Figure 1.1 represents a move towards an integrated theoretical prospective in understanding and approaching dementia.

Dementia is a condition that can be understood from biomedical, psychosocial and gerontological vantage points.

Dementia research will focus on macro and micro level issues to promote a broader understanding of the worlds of professionals, carers and people with dementia. This would be contextualised within policy frameworks and societal expectations and beliefs about dementia and quality care.

Policy frameworks need to reflect biomedical knowledge and psychosocial concerns about the individual, while recognising the disadvantage(s) older people face in society.

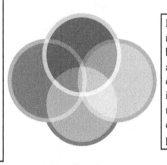

Care practices need to take account of individuals and their neurological impairment, while taking account of the structural constraints in providing high quality care.

Figure 1.1 A web of understanding dementia using an integrated perspective

Linking theory and policy: an integrated approach?

This chapter has highlighted the implications of different theoretical starting points and perspectives about dementia for the approach to dementia policy, practice and research. There are, of course, wider ramifications for understanding, questioning and furthering knowledge on particular conditions from different theoretical starting points. For example, Prior (2003) has highlighted a movement generally for patients, rather than professional paid workers to be seen as 'experts'. Deciding whose account to listen to and to act on will have huge implications for the care services that are offered and the manner in which they are delivered.

The key message of this chapter is that theory matters; conceptualisation(s) of a condition has significant ramifications for those diagnosed or labelled with that condition. Dementia has afforded discussions presented as a series of paradoxes and polarisations within contemporary debates. A tendency to critique models of care based on their theoretical origins, while necessary to advance our thinking, has perhaps been an obstacle to the development of models that embrace the positive contribution that each theory can make to understanding how best to support and care for people with dementia, and to developing actionable policy with clear implementation plans. However, critiques have contributed much to the field, particularly in relation to diagnosis and by offering suggestions for the prevention of risk from developing dementia in the future.

Social psychological perspectives have offered insights into the interventions and support that can be offered to people with dementia, but they also highlight the individual with a dementia diagnosis; the problem with psychological perspectives, as we have seen, is overemphasis on the individual and the need to improve individual care practices. This has meant that there have not been universal improvements in dementia care practices. Social gerontological perspectives alert us to the importance of recognising both wider social structures and the influence these have on individuals' experiences. We need to acknowledge and use the knowledge we have gained from different perspectives to bring about progress in the field of dementia services and continue to improve the lives of people with dementia.

Conclusion

This chapter has provided a critical assessment of different theoretical perspectives from a social science standpoint. For a truly integrated dementia care model to evolve, the lessons from different theoretical perspectives need to be explicitly recognised, challenged and valued. Doing this would help to substantiate the rhetoric of holistic models by underpinning it with a wider conceptual basis that promotes genuine holistic practice, instead of paying lip service to such approaches while persisting in a traditional pattern of delivering care.

References

Age Concern England (2007) *Improving Services and Support for Older People with Mental Health Problems.* London: Age Concern England. Available at www.ageconcern.org.uk/AgeConcern/Documents/fullreport.pdf

Alzheimer Europe (2008) 'Europe unites against Alzheimer's disease.' *Dementia in Europe 2*, 22–26.

Alzheimer Society (2011) *Demography.* Available at http://alzheimers.org.uk/site/scripts/documents_info.php?documentID=412

Alzheimer's Disease International (2010) *Statistics.* Available at www.alz.co.uk/research/statistics.html

Bond, J. (1992) 'The medicalization of dementia.' *Journal of Aging Studies 4*, 397–403.

Clare, L. (2003) 'Managing threats to self: awareness in early stage Alzheimer's disease.' *Social Science and Medicine 57*, 6, 1017–1029.

Clare, L. (2004) 'Awareness in early-stage Alzheimer's disease: a review of methods and evidence.' *British Journal of Clinical Psychology 43*, 2, 177–196.

Cowdell, F. (2006) 'Preserving personhood in dementia research: a literature review.' *International Journal of Older People Nursing 1*, 2, 85–94.

Crisp, A.H., Gelder, M.G., Rix, S., Meltzer, H.I. and Rowlands, O.J. (2000) 'Stigmatisation of people with mental illnesses.' *The British Journal of Psychiatry 177*, 1, 4–7.

Department of Health (2009) *Living Well with Dementia: A National Dementia Strategy*. London: Department of Health.

Department of Health and Social Security and Public Safety (DHSSPS) (2010) *Improving Dementia Services in Northern Ireland: A Regional Strategy*. Available at www.dhsspsni.gov.uk/improving-dementia-services-in-northern-ireland-consultation-may-2010.pdf

Devlin, E., MacAskill, S. and Stead, M. (2007) '"We're still the same people": developing a mass media campaign to raise awareness and challenge the stigma of dementia.' *International Journal of Nonprofit and Voluntary Sector Marketing 12*, 1, 47–58.

Dewing, J. (2008) 'Personhood and dementia: revisiting Tom Kitwood's ideas.' *International Journal of Older People Nursing 3*, 3–13.

Dillman, R.J.M. (2000) 'Alzheimer Disease: Epistemological Lessons from History?' In P.J. Whitehouse, K. Maurer and J.F. Ballenger (eds) *Concepts of Alzheimer Disease: Biological, Clinical and Cultural Perspectives*. Baltimore: Johns Hopkins University Press.

Dressel, P., Minkler, M. and Yen, I. (1997) 'Gender, race, class and aging: advances and opportunities.' *International Journal of Health Services 27*, 4, 579–600.

Edvardsson, D., Winblad, B. and Sandman, P.O. (2008) 'Person-centred care of people with severe Alzheimer's disease: current status and ways forward.' *Lancet Neurology 7*, 362–367.

Estes, C.L., Biggs, S. and Phillipson, C. (2003) *Social Theory, Social Policy and Ageing: A Critical Introduction*. Buckingham: Open University Press.

European Parliament (2011) *European Parliament Resolution of 19 January 2011 on a European Initiative on Alzheimer's Disease and Other Dementias*. Available at www.europarl.europa.eu/sides/getDoc. do?type=TA&reference=P7-TA-2011-0016&language=EN

Fox, P.J. (2000) 'The Role of the Concept of Alzheimer Disease in the Development of the Alzheimer's Association in the United States.' In P.J. Whitehouse, K. Maurer and J.F. Ballenger (eds) *Concepts of Alzheimer Disease: Biological, Clinical and Cultural Perspectives*. Baltimore: Johns Hopkins University Press.

Goffman, G.E. (1963) *Stigma: Notes on the Management of Spoiled Identity*. Englewood Cliffs, NY: Prentice Hall.

Goldsmith, M. (1996) *Hearing the Voice of People with Dementia*. London: Jessica Kingsley Publishers.

Gubrium, J.F. (1986) *Old Timers and Alzheimer's: The Descriptive Organization of Senility*. Greenwich: JAI Press.

Harding, N. and Palfrey, C. (1997) *The Social Construction of Dementia: Confused Professionals?* London: Jessica Kingsley Publishers.

Harris, P.B. (2008) 'Another wrinkle in the debate about successful aging: the undervalued concept of resilience and the lived experience of dementia.' *International Journal of Aging and Human Development 67*, 1, 43–61.

Harris, P.B. and Keady, J. (2008) 'Wisdom, resilience and successful aging: changing public discourses on living with dementia.' *Dementia 7*, 1, 5–8.

Holstein, M. (1997) 'Alzheimer's disease and senile dementia, 1885–1920: an interpretive history of disease negotiation.' *Journal of Aging Studies 11*, 1, 1–13.

Hughes, J.C. (2011) *Thinking through Dementia*. Oxford: Oxford University Press.

Hulko, W. (2004) 'Social Science Perspectives on Dementia Research: Intersectionality.' In A. Innes, C. Archibald and C. Murphy (eds) *Dementia and Social Inclusion: Marginalised Groups and Marginalised Areas of Dementia Research, Care and Practice*. London: Jessica Kingsley Publishers.

Innes, A. (2002) 'The social and political context of formal dementia provision.' *Ageing and Society 22*, 483–499.

Innes, A. (2009) *Dementia Studies: A Social Science Perspective*. London: Sage.

Innes, A., Macpherson, S. and McCabe, L. (2006) *Promoting Person-Centred Care at the Frontline*. York: Joseph Rowntree Foundation. Available at www.jrf.org.uk/bookshop/eBooks/9781859354520.pdf

Innes, A., Sleator, H., Kelly, F., Egner, A. and McManus, M. (2010) *Consultation Exercise for Dementia Users and Carers.* Available at www.dhsspsni.gov.uk/dsdc-report-consultation-exercise-for-dementia-users-and-carers.pdf

Kelly, F. (2010) 'Recognising and supporting self in dementia: a new way to facilitate a person-centred approach to dementia care.' *Ageing and Society 30,* 1, 103–124.

Kitwood, T. (1990) 'The dialectics of dementia, with particular reference to Alzheimer's disease.' *Ageing and Society 10,* 2, 177–196.

Kitwood, T. (1993) 'Towards a theory of dementia care: the interpersonal process.' *Ageing and Society 13,* 51–67.

Kitwood, T. (1997) *Dementia Reconsidered: The Person Comes First.* Buckingham: Open University Press.

Knapp, M., Prince, M., Albanese, E., Banerjee, S. *et al.* (2007) *Dementia UK.* London: Alzheimer Society. Available at http://alzheimers.org.uk/site/scripts/download_info.php?fileID=2

Lyman, K.A. (1989) 'Bringing the social back in: a critique of the bio-medicalisation of dementia.' *The Gerontologist 29,* 5, 597–604.

McCormack, B. (2004) 'Person-centredness in gerontological nursing: an overview of the literature.' *International Journal of Older People Nursing 13,* 31–38.

National Audit Office (2007) *Improving Services and Support for People with Dementia.* London: Stationery Office.

Parker, J. (2005) 'Constructing dementia and dementia care: daily practices in a day care setting.' *Journal of Social Work 5,* 261–278.

Poveda, A.M. (2003) 'An anthropological perspective of Alzheimer disease.' *Geriatric Nursing 24,* 1, 26–31.

Prior, L. (2003) 'Belief, knowledge and expertise: the emergence of the lay expert in medical sociology.' *Sociology of Health and Illness 25,* 41–57.

Sabat, S. (2002) 'Surviving manifestations of selfhood in Alzheimer's disease: a case study.' *Dementia 1,* 1, 25–36.

Sabat, S. and Harré, R. (1992) 'The construction and deconstruction of self in Alzheimer's disease.' *Ageing and Society 12,* 4, 443–461.

Sabat, S.R. (1994) 'Excess disability and malignant social-psychology – a case study of Alzheimer's disease.' *Journal of Community and Applied Social Psychology 4,* 3, 157–166.

Sabat, S.R. (2001) *The Experience of Alzheimer's Disease: Life through a Tangled Veil.* Oxford: Blackwell.

Sabat, S.R. (2006) 'Mind, Meaning and Personhood in Dementia: The Effects of Positioning.' In J.C. Hughes, S.J. Louw and S.R. Sabat (eds) *Dementia: Mind, Meaning and the Person.* Oxford: Oxford University Press.

Scottish Government (2010) *Scotland's National Dementia Strategy.* Available at www.scotland.gov.uk/Publications/2010/09/10151751/0

Walker, A. and Phillipson, C. (1986) *Ageing and Social Policy: A Critical Assessment.* Aldershot: Gower.

Wilson, G. and Fearnley, K. (2007) *The Dementia Epidemic – Where Scotland is Now and the Challenge Ahead.* Edinburgh: Alzheimer Scotland.

Chapter 2

Developing Evidence for Action

DEMENTIA CARE IN CANADA

Scott Dudgeon

The context

In 2006 it was clear that the Alzheimer Society of Canada (ASC) needed a re-focused approach to advocacy. Having just assumed my role as ASC's Chief Executive Officer after having led a national project to strengthen mental health care, I believed that the people who set priorities for government didn't fully understand the total impact of either mental health issues generally, or dementia specifically, on society. Furthermore, I believed that with such understanding they would be more inclined to act. I soon came to the view that we would need to work hard to help government see that it is important for them to take coordinated action on what the scientists had explained to me is a very serious epidemic.

The Alzheimer Society was already adept at marshalling the voices of people with dementia and their caregivers, but it was clear that we needed to balance the emotive argument with a rational analysis built upon an up-to-date understanding of the scale of dementia in Canada. Our advocacy efforts to date had relied upon findings from the Canadian Study of Health and Aging, a landmark study of the epidemiology of Alzheimer's Disease and related dementias published in 1994. This goldmine of epidemiological information was the basis of how dementia was viewed by government, by the research community and by the Alzheimer Society. However, we were concerned that, notwithstanding its excellence, much had happened in the intervening years to change the cost structure of the disease and to further our understanding of the nature of the challenge. A fresh approach was called for.

We decided to develop an advocacy document, *Rising Tide: The Impact of Dementia in Canada* (Alzheimer Society of Canada 2009), a synthesis of the epidemiology and economic impact of dementia, the development of policy options based on a review of international responses to the dementia epidemic, evaluation of the potential savings that would accrue from selected intervention scenarios, and a recommended course of action for governments. The impact of this approach far exceeded our best hopes.

The Canadian cancer community had made impressive gains in securing significant Federal funding, largely on the strength of a business case prepared by RiskAnalytica, a decision analysis consultancy in Toronto, using its simulation platform to assess the population health and economic impacts of cancer in Canada. We engaged RiskAnalytica to provide the analytical basis for the advocacy case which the Alzheimer Society would make. We needed to identify how many people in Canada had dementia and to assess what was then the current economic impact (2008). Because dementia is in the early phases of an epidemic, we also thought it would be prudent to forecast the prevalence and economic impact in 2038 – roughly a generation later.

Phase I: the base case

In order to quantify the expected impact of the dementia epidemic on Canadian society, we recruited and collaborated with a wide range of dementia subject matter experts (people with dementia, caregivers, psychiatrists, neurologists, geriatricians, long-term care managers, nurses, social workers, and Alzheimer Society staff) in order to get a clear sense of the various journeys that may be taken by individuals with dementia. Together, we diagrammed the disease management process – the journey for individuals with dementia from the existence of risk factors to appearance of symptoms, diagnosis, treatment, care at home and in the community, long-term care, and end-of-life care. It became clear as we mapped the journey that the family caregiver is a vital part of the picture throughout the process, from beginning to end.

We next asked our team of experts to help us find peer-reviewed journal articles that would illuminate such key data elements as number of caregiver hours at each phase of the illness, length of time from diagnosis to initiation of treatment, and so on, to form the statistical basis for modeling the economic impact of the disease. At the time these conversations were taking place, there was quite a bit of discussion in the research community about the role of a diverse range of risk and protective factors, but we could find no research evidence that would cause us to reflect these in our statistical assumptions. We searched widely to identify more recent epidemiological approaches than the Canadian Study of Health and Aging (Canadian Medical Association 1994). While we incorporated learning from the EURODEM pooled analyses, which explored the prevalence of dementia in the elderly in Europe (Berr, Wancata and Ritchie 2005), the Canadian Study formed the primary epidemiological basis. Cost drivers for the economic analysis were derived from the research literature, and basic population and economic data were taken from the most recent Statistics Canada statistical databases.

After customizing the simulation platform to reflect the key epidemiological and economic assumptions related to dementia, RiskAnalytica ran it to establish the base case, a forecast of the population health and economic impact of dementia on Canadian society each year, for the next 30 years. The base case assumes no change in policy, no new scientific discovery and no intervention. The resultant profile includes measures of population health and economic burden attributable to dementia.

By simulating anticipated population changes and evidence-based assumptions about dementia between 2008 and 2058, we were able to forecast, for each year, the number of expected new dementia cases (incidence) and deaths (mortality), as well as how many people in Canada we can expect to be living with dementia (prevalence), assuming no policy or other intervention.

Finally, by applying research-based assumptions for direct, indirect and opportunity costs, we are able to forecast the total cost associated with dementia (economic burden), both on an annual basis in future dollars (adjusted for inflation) 10, 20 and 30 years into the future, and on a cumulative basis for 10, 20 and 30 years as present values in 2008 dollars. Together, these dimensions illustrate the base case burden of dementia in Canada, expressed both as discrete values and as confidence intervals.

Base case: major findings

INCIDENCE

- Projected incidence:
  - ○ 2008: 104,000 new dementia cases per year.
  - ○ 2038: 258,000 new dementia cases per year.

PREVALENCE

- The number of Canadians (of all ages) with dementia is expected to increase to 2.3 times the current level to 1.1 million people by 2038, representing 2.8 per cent of the Canadian population. Projected prevalence:
  - ○ 2008: 481,000 people, or 1.5 per cent of the Canadian population.
  - ○ 2038: 1,125,000 people, or 2.8 per cent of the Canadian population.

- Persons with Alzheimer's disease (AD) and vascular dementia (VD) will account for the vast majority of dementia cases in Canada (approximately 83%):

  o 2008: 304,000 cases (63%) AD / 94,000 (19.5%) VD.

  o 2038: 771,000 cases (69.5%) AD / 221,000 (20%) VD.

- The prevalence of dementia is higher in females than males, with a ratio of approximately 1.36 throughout the simulation period.

  o The average female to male ratio of AD prevalence is approximately 2.3.

  o The average female to male ratio of VD prevalence is approximately 0.85.

- The proportion of the Canadian population who have dementia increases with age. The percentage of Canadians with dementia is projected as:

  o 2008: 7 per cent of Canadians over age 60 are expected to have dementia; 49 per cent of Canadians over age 90 are expected to have dementia.

  o 2038: 9 per cent of Canadians over age 60 are expected to have dementia; 50 per cent of Canadians over age 90 are expected to have dementia.

- Prevalence of dementia in Canada is expected to skew toward the older age groups due to general aging of the Canadian population. The expected increase in the percentage of people with dementia who are over the age of 80 is as follows:

  o *In total*. 2008: 60 per cent of people with dementia are over age 80; 2038: 73 per cent of people with dementia are forecasted to be over age 80.

  o *AD*. 2008: 71 per cent of people with AD are over age 80; 2038: 78 per cent of people with AD are forecasted to be over age 80.

  o *VD*. 2008: 51 per cent of people with VD are over age 80; 2038: 61 per cent of people with VD are forecasted to be over age 80.

CARE SETTINGS

By categorizing those living with dementia according to the type and location of care which research evidence suggests that they will be receiving, and by applying expected long-term care capacity constraints, we were able to form a profile of care delivery – a picture of how and where care will be provided – to people living with dementia.

Dementia prevalence increases across all care types over the 30-year simulation period. However, there is a significant shift from institutional care toward home/community-based care.

- In 2008, 55 per cent of individuals over age 65 with dementia were living in their own homes, most with the support of some kind of community care (CC).

- By 2038, 63 per cent of individuals over age 65 with dementia are expected to be living in their own homes. This represents an increase of 510,000 people and would substantially increase CC and caregiver burden.

The task of caregiving changes throughout the progression of dementia. Initially, when the person with dementia is still living at home, the focus for the informal caregiver may be on helping with transportation, household finance, meals and day-to-day living activities. By the time the individual is receiving care at home from community service providers, the scope of the caregiving role broadens to include supervision to ensure safety. Once the individual is in a nursing home, the needs change again. While support for activities of daily living is provided by the care facility, the caregiver continues to be engaged as a member of the care team to provide supportive care, including social engagement and affection.

- By 2038, the total number of hours of informal care (family and friends) is expected to more than triple, increasing from approximately 231 million hours in 2008, to 756 million hours.

- Informal caregivers within community care settings account for the largest proportion of informal care, increasing from 60 per cent to 69 per cent over the 30-year simulation period.

Economic impact

The study's economic framework calculated the total expected economic burden of dementia as the sum of direct health costs, opportunity costs (foregone wages) of unpaid family caregivers, and indirect costs. *Direct health costs* are costs incurred for treating and providing care to individuals with dementia. Direct health costs pertaining to dementia include the cost of medication, long-term care costs, and physician and hospital costs.

Opportunity costs of family caregivers are the wages that could be earned by family caregivers, were they able to participate in the labour force. *Indirect costs* reflect lost production and corporate profits – costs that have no direct connection to health care, but are a consequence of dementia.

Expected annual total economic burden, expressed in future dollars,[1] increases substantially from approximately $15 billion in 2008 to $153 billion by 2038. Approximately one-third of the economic burden is borne by family caregivers.

- The monetary burden of dementia (direct plus indirect costs) is expected to reach approximately $97 billion by 2038.

- Opportunity costs of informal caregivers are expected to add a further $56 billion to the annual economic burden by 2038.

Base case: conclusions

Since age is a primary and immutable risk factor for dementia, the growth of the dementia problem in Canada will accelerate as the population ages. We know that the first of the baby boomers will enter their senior years in the next couple of years, at which time the aging of the Canadian population will accelerate. This will place a tremendous strain on the capacity of Canada's health care systems to provide essential health care services and community care as well as patient and caregiver support services, potentially overwhelming the Canadian health care system.

The results of the Rising Tide project show that without intervention:

- By 2038 the rate of dementia incidence is expected to increase to 250,000 new cases per year, 2.5 times the current level (2008). By 2038 1.1 million Canadians are expected to have dementia, approximately 2.8 per cent of all Canadians and 9 per cent of Canadians over 60.

- Over the next 30 years, dementia is expected to cost Canadian society an accumulated $872 billion dollars in direct health costs, unpaid caregiver opportunity costs and indirect costs associated with the provision of unpaid care.

---

1   The simulation model provides results both on an annual basis in future dollars (adjusted for inflation) 10, 20 and 30 years into the future, and on a cumulative basis for 10, 20 and 30 years as present values in 2008 dollars.

Phase II: scenario analysis

The first phase of the Rising Tide project established a base case: what would happen if the dementia epidemic proceeded unimpeded by any major change in policy? However disturbing the results are, the intent of the base case is not just to alarm. It is intended to evoke a call to action, and it is intended to be the line in the sand against which we evaluate our ability to take meaningful action that will change the course of the base case, whether by reducing dementia incidence, or by bending the cost curve.

In the scenario analysis phase of the Rising Tide project, we assessed how targeted interventions could reduce the burden of dementia. Four intervention scenarios were generated, representing potential dementia prevention and patient/caregiver support programs. The selected scenarios are not meant to be the final word on what must be done. They are meant to illustrate how, using either evidence or hypothesis, policy options can be evaluated and compared in a very practical way.

Selection of the four intervention scenarios depended not only upon the anticipated health and economic value of the interventions, but also on the availability of evidence-based data to support the simulations. Intervention scenario results are expressed in 'value' terms – that is, in terms of how each intervention would *change* the health and economic burden of dementia in Canada. The cost of achieving these benefits was not identified; the intent was to focus and support consideration of investment alternatives: 'What would we be prepared to spend to achieve a benefit of x?'

The outcomes of the proposed dementia intervention scenarios were compared to the base case to derive the expected relative value of the interventions. The value analysis for each of the scenarios is summarized below.

The scenarios

INTERVENTION 1: PREVENTION – INCREASE IN PHYSICAL ACTIVITY

The first prevention scenario examines the impact of an intervention which broadly applies evidence that increased physical activity may reduce dementia incidence. The intervention focuses on increasing physical activity by 50 per cent for all Canadians without dementia who are over the age of 65 and who already rate themselves as moderately to highly active. Such intervention has been shown to significantly reduce the number of people diagnosed with dementia in the short and long term.

Supporting data were derived from the Statistics Canada CANSIM database and the odds ratios related to physical activity from the Canadian Study of Health and Aging (Laurin *et al.* 2001).

The follow-on effects of this reduction result in fewer people living with dementia and a reduction in the pressure on long-term care, community care and informal care. This, in turn, was shown to produce significant savings in direct health costs, unpaid caregiver opportunity costs and indirect costs associated with dementia and the provision of care by informal caregivers throughout the simulation timeframe.

Intervention 2: prevention – a program
to delay dementia onset

The second intervention scenario examines the impact of a hypothetical prevention program which would delay the onset of dementia by approximately two years. The prevention program targets the entire dementia-free adult Canadian population and would combine a variety of promising, evidence-based strategies such as following a healthy diet and lifestyle.

A comprehensive study by Brookmeyer *et al.* (2007) estimates that the relative (expected) effect of such a prevention program would translate into a 23 per cent drop in overall annual incidence. This scenario assumes that the relative risk factor is equally applicable across all dementia disease types, both genders and all age groups (65+).

Relative to the base case, delaying the onset of dementia by two years resulted in fewer people living with dementia and significantly reduced the constraints placed on health care resources and the health care system. This intervention was shown to produce significant savings in health costs, informal caregiver opportunity costs and indirect costs associated with dementia and informal care throughout the simulated timeframe.

Intervention 3: support – caregiver
development and support program

This scenario examines the impact of an informal caregiver skill-building and support program. Such a program could reduce the amount of caregiving time and hence the health and economic burden placed on informal caregivers. As well, it could delay admission for the person with dementia into long-term care. In this scenario the intervention is applied to all informal caregivers and individuals with dementia receiving care within the model.

The reduction in caregiving time from such a program is based on a study by Graff *et al.* (2008). The study showed that informal caregiver hours could be reduced by an average of 212.3 hours over a three-month timeframe by providing a program of occupational therapy to patients and their informal caregivers targeting improvement in:

- informal caregiver competence, skills and communications strategies for supervision of activities of daily living

- coping strategies for patient behaviours and the overall burden of care.

An informal caregiver support program has also been shown to delay patient admissions into long-term care. These effects are based on a study by Mittelman *et al.* (2006). This study showed that long-term care placement could be delayed for dementia patients by a median of 557 days by providing a counselling and support intervention program for spousal caregivers. This scenario therefore assumes that individuals who would have been admitted to long-term care under the base case (no intervention) scenario will do so after a 557-day delay. It further assumes that the impact on all types of informal caregivers parallels that of the spouses in the study.

Intervention 4: support – system navigator

The fourth scenario examines the impact of assigning a system navigator (case manager) to each newly diagnosed dementia patient in order to provide care coordination to people with dementia and caregiver support to informal caregivers. In this scenario the intervention is for all people with dementia and their informal caregivers.

The effects of a system navigator are modeled on the Lewisham Case Management Scheme from a study by Challis *et al.* (2002). This study showed that individuals with dementia and their caregivers who received an intensive case management service remained in the community longer, had a reduced informal caregiver burden and had reduced overall costs relative to those receiving usual care. The study concluded that a system navigator would delay long-term care admission by two years and would reduce informal caregiving hours.

It is anticipated that providing a system navigator would delay admission into long-term care and that this would reduce the pressure placed on long-term care resources, producing significant savings in health costs. Delaying admission into long-term care is expected to result in more people with dementia relying on community-based care and informal care resources.

As in Intervention 3, provision of a system navigator is anticipated to reduce the economic burden on informal caregivers. As compared to the base model, this is expected to produce significant savings in informal caregiver opportunity costs as well as the indirect costs associated with informal care provision throughout the simulated timeframe.

Scenario analysis: conclusions

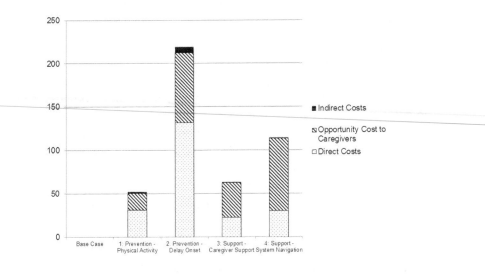

Figure 2.1 Cumulative 30-year savings impact of interventions on total
economic burden (2008; dollars) (Alzheimer Society of Canada 2009)

The intervention scenarios demonstrate the following points, which are
represented in graph form in Figure 2.1 above:

- Increasing the activity level of seniors who are already active
  (Intervention 1) would yield a 30-year reduction in direct health costs
  of $31 billion and a reduction in total economic burden of $52 billion.

- Delaying onset of dementia by two years (Intervention 2) would yield
  a 30-year reduction of $219 billion in total economic burden, along
  with a reduction in prevalence of 410,000 individuals – a 36 per cent
  reduction from the base case.

- Helping caregivers develop coping skills and build competencies in
  their caregiving roles (Intervention 3) would yield a 30-year value of
  $63 billion.

- Providing system navigation support to people with dementia and
  their caregivers (Intervention 4) would yield a 30-year value of $114
  billion.

- Each of the four scenarios delivers significant value, indicating clearly
  that efforts to devise an intervention or suite of interventions, with the
  goal of substantially delaying onset of dementia, warrant attention.

- The Rising Tide approach and RiskAnalytica's modeling platform together provide a useful assessment and comparison methodology for conducting evidence-based strategic options and policy analysis.

Phase III: policy analysis

The final phase of the Rising Tide project involved looking at existing and emerging policy responses to the dementia epidemic in other countries and in different parts of Canada. This review was not meant to be encyclopedic; it was meant to reveal a rich range of options for the consideration of the Alzheimer Society and Canada's policy makers. The analysis concludes with recommendations for consideration. These recommendations, if adopted by policy makers and decision makers in Canada, will cause fewer people to die with dementia and will reduce the disease's impact on Canadian society.

What has been done in other countries?

There are more than 35 million people with dementia in the world at this time. It is estimated that by 2050 this number will increase to 115 million people (Alzheimer's Disease International 2009). Owing to a number of factors – ageism, stigma associated with mental disorders, recency of treatment options – the policy response has been dismal in most countries, with a few notable exceptions.

Australia, Norway, the Netherlands, Scotland, France and England have each developed specific plans or frameworks for dealing with dementia, largely directed at greater integration of health and social policies: establishing more home-based programming, adapting care facilities to better meet the needs of residents with dementia, education for people with dementia, their families, health professionals and the public, and investment in research. In 2008, the Council of the European Union passed a number of resolutions committing the European Parliament to support European action to combat neurodegenerative diseases, particularly Alzheimer's disease.

The dementia-specific policies of six countries that have made dementia a health priority were reviewed by the Alzheimer Society and are summarized in Table 2.1. Each offers valuable lessons for thinking about Canada's needs.

There are several common elements. All of the strategies are recent. Most acknowledge the importance of investing in research, supporting caregivers in their role and improving the skills of professionals who provide care to people with dementia. Strategies to improve the delivery of care to people with dementia include focusing on early diagnosis and intervention, use of case management, specialized home care, and making information about the disease widely available through channels such as telecare.

A comparison of national dementia strategies also highlights some unique features:

- the call for a national priority in the United Kingdom with cross-government strategy development
- the notion of Alzheimer holidays, hotels and farms in the Netherlands
- the Dutch concept of building the national strategy on the foundation of problems identified, experienced and prioritized by people with dementia and their caregivers
- the French concept of mobilizing society for the fight against dementia
- the French goal of making dementia a European priority.

What has been tried in Canada?

Health care in Canada is primarily the responsibility of the provinces and territories. The role of the Federal Government of Canada in the provision of health services is limited to specified populations, namely First Nations and Inuit, members of the Canadian Armed Forces, veterans, federal public servants working abroad and inmates of federal correctional facilities. The Federal Government's most significant role in provision for dementia is the funding of dementia research, primarily through the Institute of Aging of Canadian Institutes of Health Research (CIHR).

As in many countries, progress in policy development is impeded by lack of clarity as to which department, among various levels of government and within each level, is to take responsibility for dementia policy. Should it be the department responsible for seniors' issues? For chronic diseases? For mental health? As a consequence, policy for the management of dementia is a disparate hodge-podge.

No government in Canada has a department that deals strictly with dementia. Each jurisdiction has found its own way to deal with the management of dementia, whether through mental health policy, their seniors' department, long-term care or chronic disease management. Most provinces and territories have policies in respect of long-term care facilities, respite care and other publicly funded or administered services used by people with dementia. The few dementia-specific strategies/policies are described below. So far, only Ontario has attached significant funding in support of strengthening dementia care in the context of provincial dementia strategies.

Canada's first comprehensive strategy on Alzheimer's disease and related dementias (ADRD) was initiated in Ontario in 1999, with $68.4 million invested in the strategy over the following five years (Ontario Government

Table 2.1 Plans for dealing with dementia in Australia, Norway, the Netherlands, Scotland, France and England

Country	Research	Improved care	Caregiver support	Workforce
Australia (2006–2010), $320 million allocated[1]	• Collaborative research centres • Additional funding • Prevention focus	• Primary care guidelines • Expanded psychogeriatric consultations • Early intervention • Helpline • Memory community centres	• Training • Home care support for behaviour problems	• Training
Norway (2006–2015)[2]	• Quality development	• Day programs • Adapted living facilities	• Partnerships with providers, families and communities	• Raising skills and knowledge • Improving collaboration among professionals • National standard to improve medical services in nursing homes
Netherlands (2008–2011)[3]		• Case management • Transportation to care settings • Peer support (Alzheimer café) • Helpline • Care hotel • Cluster housing with home automation	• Client/person-centred policy development • Respite, temporary stays, holidays	
Scotland (2008–2011)[4]	• Enhance research funding • Network	• Early diagnosis, intervention • Post-diagnostic support • Integration of palliative care	• Information	

France (2008–2012), €1.6 billion allocated[5]	• Partnerships, network	• Integrated access points • 1000 case managers • In-home specialist teams • Telephone hotline	• Respite care • Strengthen caregiver rights, education, support for return to work • Improve health monitoring of caregivers	• Developing skill sets in all care professionals • Develop new competencies – case managers, gerontology assistants
England (2009–2013), £150 million allocated[6]	• Increase funding for dementia care research	• Early diagnosis and intervention • Public information to promote help-seeking • Easy access to care • Peer support • Specialist home care services • Improved care for people with dementia in general hospitals • Housing support • Telecare • Improved end-of-life care • Develop comprehensive model of care	• Information • Carer needs assessment • Carer strategy	• Training, continuing professional development in dementia for care professionals

1 Australian Health Ministers' Conference, National Framework for Action on Dementia 2006–2011, www.health.gov.au/internet/main/publishing.nsf/Content/B96166 04C02332D5CA25701B0075A997/$File/NFAD%20low%20res%20Web%20Version%20Oct%2006.pdf, 2006.

2 Norwegian Ministry of Health and Care Services, Dementia Plan 2015, www.regjeringen.no/upload/HOD/Dokumenter%20KTA/DementiaPlan2015.pdf, 2008.

3 State Secretary for Health, Welfare and Sports, Dutch Dementia Care Plan, www.alzheimer-europe.org/Policy-in-Practice2/National-Dementia-Plans/Netherlands, 2008.

4 The Scottish Government, Scotland's National Dementia Strategy, www.scotland.gov.uk/Resource/Doc/324377/0104420.pdf, 2010.

5 Alzheimer Europe, National Plan for 'Alzheimer and Related Diseases': 2008–2012, www.alzheimer-europe.org/Policy-in-Practice2/National-Dementia-Plans/France, 2008.

6 Department of Health, Living Well with Dementia: A National Dementia Strategy, www.dh.gov.uk/prod_consum_dh/groups/dh_digitalassets/@dh/@en/documents/digitalasset/dh_094051.pdf, 2009.

2005). The strategy, under the auspices of the Ministry of Health and Long-Term Care and the Seniors' Secretariat of the Ministry of Citizenship and Immigration, comprised ten initiatives:

1. Staff education and training.
2. Physician training.
3. Increase public awareness, information and education.
4. Planning for appropriate, safe and secure environments.
5. Respite services for caregivers.
6. Research on caregiver needs.
7. Advance directives on care choices.
8. Psychogeriatric consulting resources.
9. Dementia networks, research coalition, specialized geriatric services.
10. Intergenerational volunteer initiative.

(Ontario Government 2005, pp.2–5)

Since the implementation of the strategy, the Ontario Government has funded the establishment of the Alzheimer Knowledge Exchange (AKE) which is a clearing house for current knowledge regarding Alzheimer's disease and related dementias, along with a resource for e-learning and web-based support for knowledge exchange. As well, services to people with dementia are being improved through the province's *Aging at Home Strategy*, a $1.1 billion (over four years) initiative designed to allow seniors to live healthy, independent lives in the comfort and dignity of their own homes.[2]

The Quebec Government has announced that it will be implementing recommendations from *Relever le défi de la maladie d'Alzheimer et des maladies apparentée*, an action plan developed by a panel of experts led by Dr Howard Bergman (2009). The expert panel recommended that the Ministry of Health and Social Services implement the recommendations over six years. Quebec's current priorities under their action plan for 2010–2015 include chronic conditions. The expert panel recommends that dementia be regarded as a chronic condition and be integrated into the ministerial action plan.

The recommendations are made in the context of significant health system reform in Quebec, including the creation of integrated services delivered through health and social service centres, along with family medicine groups and clinical networks.

---

2   See www.health.gov.on.ca/english/public/program/ltc/34_strategy_Qa.html#1

The plan defines seven priority actions, incorporating 24 recommendations:

1. Raise awareness, inform and mobilize.

2. Ensure the availability of locally responsive, personalized and coordinated services and evidence-based treatment for people with dementia and their caregivers.

3. In advanced stages of the disease, promote quality of life and provide access to home support.

4. Promote quality end-of-life care, in accordance with the wishes of the client and family, and characterized by dignity and comfort.

5. Provide services to family caregivers: partners in support.

6. Develop and support professional practice.

7. Mobilize an unprecedented research effort.

As of 2011, this widely hailed plan has not been resourced.

A review of dementia strategies from several countries and several Canadian provinces reveals general agreement on key elements in any comprehensive dementia strategy:

- The public needs better access to information to increase awareness, to overcome stigma, and to seek help, so that early interventions can be initiated.

- Health professionals who provide care to individuals with dementia need to be supported in their knowledge needs to ensure that dementia is recognized and that the professionals know what treatments and care strategies are appropriate for different stages in the disease.

- Helping caregivers cope, reducing the financial disincentives to fulfill caregiving roles and ensuring that caregivers are supported with respite and training are critical features.

- Case management and system navigation are becoming important features of dementia strategies.

- Organizing services along the lines of the chronic disease prevention and management model is congruent with current policy direction in several provinces.

- Continued investment in research is a common feature.

The impact of Rising Tide

There has been tremendous public response to the Society's advocacy document, *Rising Tide: The Impact of Dementia in Canada* (Alzheimer Society of Canada 2009).

Prior to running the base case, we released preliminary prevalence data which were limited to Canadians 65 years and older, due to the fact the epidemiological studies we used, and those used by others, did not count people under 65. However, this bias was at odds with our own experience. We were meeting people all across the country who had been diagnosed with Alzheimer's disease or some other dementia in their fifties or earlier. It was difficult for these individuals to get a diagnosis when clinicians were conditioned to see these diseases as relevant only to older people. This difficulty was compounded by the incredulity of friends and family, who had trouble accepting that such a diagnosis was possible. Therefore, with the help of expert epidemiologists, we extrapolated backward the age-specific prevalence rates to derive an under-65 prevalence of approximately 70,000 individuals. When speaking of this number, we were always quick to point out that it does not have the epidemiological rigour of the other data in our study, but it was surely far closer to the truth than the presumed zero of prior studies.

This seemingly small aspect of the study had a surprisingly profound effect. First, younger people with dementia told us that they felt validated – they no longer felt invisible. Second, because the baby boomers comprise such a large and vocal part of the Canadian population, there was tremendous media interest in this aspect of the story. Boomers who were hitherto disposed to think of dementia as a future problem had seen the possibility of worrying about their parents' brain health as somewhat proximate, but the possibility of their own dementia as remote. Now dementia seemed more real, more personal.

The reporting of the findings on current and projected prevalence was picked up by the media across the country. Interviews, in-depth stories and editorials were carried in national print and electronic media and in local media across the country.

The report was released in January 2010 and generated considerable discussion. At around the same time, and in some measure, as a consequence of Rising Tide, the collective advocacy efforts of members of the Neurological Health Charities Canada (NHCC)[3] were starting to have considerable effect in the political realm. NHCC secured a commitment from the Prime Minister

---

3   The Neurological Health Charities Canada is a coalition of 25 charitable organizations that fund research and provide support to people with neurological conditions. See www.mybrainmatters.ca/en/member-profiles.

to fund a $15 million population study to better understand the scale and impact of neurological conditions in Canada. A small number of Members of Parliament from each political party, motivated by the experience of someone with one brain condition or another in each of their families, came together to explore how they might be able to do something helpful for Canadians with neurological conditions. They formed the Subcommittee for Neurological Conditions, reporting to Parliament's Standing Committee on Health. (This was the first time this Standing Committee had formed such a condition-focused subcommittee.)

NHCC, buoyed by the success of the request for a population study and by the gathering momentum, grew in membership. The members agreed to propose to Government that the coalition be funded to develop the policy necessary to support a National Brain Strategy. Rising Tide was offered as a starting point and, with the addition of recommendations for income support and for actions to reduce discrimination on the basis of genetic endowment, formed the framework for the proposed National Brain Strategy. In the 2011 Federal election, this framework became a significant plank in the platform of the Liberal Party, the Official Opposition.

Conclusion

Canadians are proud of their health care system, often to the point of being blind to some of its more persistent weaknesses. The strength of the system is that it is an expression of the Canadian value of looking out for each other – a positive aspect of the garrison mentality that Canadian literary critics regard as a characteristic of Canadian culture. This is seen as a key differentiator when comparing our health care system with that of our neighbours to the south. We accept that there is a social good to be achieved if our health care services are universally accessible.

It is no small challenge to maintain this strength in a country whose population is distributed across a vast land. In our Canada Health Act, there is an implicit promise to make services universally accessible to residents of major cities and outposts in the far north alike. This challenge was made all the more difficult from the outset when responsibilities were distributed between provinces and the Federal Government when Canada was established. Provinces are responsible for delivering health services. The Federal Government, with a few well-circumscribed exceptions, does not. It is responsible for ensuring that the health systems operated by the provinces adhere to a few agreed-upon principles (comprehensiveness, universality, public administration, portability and accessibility). The incentive for provincial compliance is maintenance of federal transfer payments.

In the Canadian health care system (an amalgam of ten provincial systems, three territorial systems and a federal role), decisions affecting the whole constellation (e.g. strengthening the primary care sector, as was undertaken in the last decade) can only be made by consensus. Consensus is difficult to achieve in a pluralistic society where the various values, histories and ideologies take the political actors to various places in the debate – provincial isolationism, regional variation. Furthermore, consensus is difficult to achieve when the provinces usually speak of any proposed change in terms of increased federal funding. The will of the Federal Government to initiate or champion change is also limited ideologically if the government of the day has a vision of the nation shaped by a belief in provincial autonomy.

Discussions with senior politicians and senior public servants suggest that the desired change will happen if the Government's caucus insists on it. That will entail that the provincial societies and local chapters of the Alzheimer Society, along with the scientific community and other friends of the cause, are aligned in their messaging and persistent in bringing the message both to candidates seeking to represent them in the federal election and to their representatives in provincial legislatures.

References

Alzheimer's Disease International (2009) *World Alzheimer's Report. Working Paper: 2009*.

Alzheimer Society of Canada (2009) *Rising Tide: The Impact of Dementia in Canada*. Available at http://alzheimersociety.sitesystems.ca/sitecore/shell/Controls/Rich%20Text%20Editor/~/media/Files/national/pdfs/English/Advocacy/ASC_Rising%20Tide_Full%20Report_Eng.ashx

Bergman, H. (2009) *Relever le défi de la maladie d'Alzheimer et des maladies apparentées*. Ministère de la Santé et des Services sociaux du Québec. Available at http://publications.msss.gouv.Qc.ca/acrobat/f/documentation/2009/09-829-01W.pdf

Berr, C., Wancata, J. and Ritchie, K. (2005) 'Prevalence of dementia in the elderly in Europe.' *European Neuropsychopharmacology 15*, 463–471.

Brookmeyer, R., Johnson, E., Ziegler-Graham, K. and Arrighi, H.M. (2007) 'Forecasting the global burden of Alzheimer's disease.' *Alzheimer's and Dementia 3*, 186–191.

Canadian Medical Association (1994) 'Canadian study of health and ageing: study methods and prevalence of dementia.' *Canadian Medical Association Journal 150*, 6, 899–913.

Challis, D., von Abendorff, R., Brown, P., Chesterman, J. and Hughes, J. (2002) 'Care management, dementia care and specialist mental health services: an evaluation.' *International Journal of Geriatric Psychiatry 17*, 4, 315–325.

Graff, M.J.L., Adang, E.M.M., Vernooij-Dassen, M.J.M., Dekker, J. *et al*. (2008) 'Community occupational therapy for older patients with dementia and their caregivers: cost effectiveness study.' *British Medical Journal*, published online 2 January 2008: doi:10.1136/bmj.39408.481898.BE.

Laurin, D., Verreault, R., Lindsay, J., MacPherson, K. and Rockwood, K. (2001) 'Physical activity and risk of cognitive impairment and dementia in elderly persons.' *Archives of Neurology 58*, 3, 498–504.

Mittelman, M.S., Haley, W.E., Clay, O.J. and Roth, D.L. (2006) 'Improving caregiver well-being delays nursing home placement of patients with Alzheimer's disease.' *Neurology 67*, 1592–1599.

Ontario Government (2005) *Ontario's Strategy for Alzheimer Disease and Related Dementia*. Available at www.health.gov.on.ca/english/public/pub/ministry_reports/alz/alz_strat.pdf

Chapter 3

Epidemiology

An Overview of Current and Predicted Epidemiological Factors Shaping Dementia Care

Nicola Coley, Claudine Berr and Sandrine Andrieu

The growing burden of dementia

The EURODEM study, a meta-analysis of European population-based studies carried out in the 1990s, estimated the age-standardized prevalence of all-cause dementia in persons aged 65 years and older in Europe to be 6.4 per cent (Lobo *et al.* 2000), with Alzheimer's disease (AD) representing the most common form of dementia. Prevalence increased with age and was estimated to be 0.8 per cent in the age group 65–69 years and 28.5 per cent in the age group 90 years and older. Dementia incidence also increases with age: a pooled study of European studies estimated an incidence rate of 2.4 per 1000 person-years in the 65–69 age group compared to 70.2 per 1000 person-years in the 90+ age group (Fratiglioni *et al.* 2000).

A Delphi consensus study (Ferri *et al.* 2005) estimated that in 2001 there were 24.3 million people with dementia in the world and that this figure was expected to double every 20 years to 81.1 million by 2040. Different regions of the world are disproportionately affected by the burden of dementia: in 2001, 60 per cent of people with dementia were estimated to live in developing countries, while by 2040 this proportion is set to rise to 71 per cent. Indeed, the rates of increase in the number of dementia cases are not uniform across regions, since the numbers in developed countries are set to increase by 100 per cent between 2001 and 2040, compared to more than 300 per cent in India, China and other South Asian and Western Pacific countries. Rapid increases in the number of people living with dementia will also be seen in African and Latin American regions.

The most recent systematic review has suggested that the prevalence of dementia may be around 10 per cent higher than previously thought. It is estimated that there were 35.6 million people living with dementia in 2010, rising to 115.4 million in 2050 (Alzheimer's Disease International 2010).

Given the increasing dependency of dementia patients, this disease places a considerable burden on patients and caregivers, as well as on society, through the use of health care resources. The estimated total worldwide cost of dementia in 2010, including informal care and formal social and medical care, was $604 billion (Alzheimer's Disease International 2010).

Risk and protective factors

Given the lack of effective treatments for dementia, attention is turning towards dementia prevention as a feasible approach for tackling this disease. The only confirmed risk factors for dementia are age, and certain genotypes, but none of these factors are modifiable. The search for modifiable risk factors is therefore one of the major focuses in aetiological epidemiological research on AD and dementia. This work is currently dominated by work assessing lifestyle-related factors such as cardiovascular risk factors or nutrition. Other factors also merit exploration, however, such as medical factors and certain environmental exposures. Some studies have assessed risk or protective factors for dementia itself, while others have assessed the effects of different factors on the rate of cognitive decline, a key feature of the dementing process.

Factors associated with chronic diseases occurring in late life can originate in earlier life stages and can accumulate over the life course (Whalley, Dick and McNeill 2006). Dementia is generally an age-associated disease, but the search for risk factors is beginning to focus not only on characteristics measured in late life just before dementia onset, but also on a more global approach taking into account the whole life course, and in particular the midlife period around 40–50 years (Fratiglioni, Paillard-Borg and Winblad 2004). Certain factors can have differential effects depending on the period of life, as, for example, has been suggested for hypertension, where it seems that high blood pressure during midlife but not late life may be a risk factor for dementia.

Below we provide a summary of the results of prospective studies that have assessed risk or protective factors for dementia or cognitive decline. Where possible, we refer to existing literature reviews or meta-analyses without covering the specific details of individual studies. The hierarchy of evidence is presented in Figure 3.1.

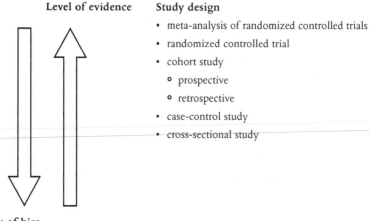

Level of evidence   Study design
- meta-analysis of randomized controlled trials
- randomized controlled trial
- cohort study
  ○ prospective
  ○ retrospective
- case-control study
- cross-sectional study

Risk of bias

Figure 3.1 Hierarchy of evidence: level of evidence and risk of bias in epidemiological studies

Sociodemographic factors

Advanced age remains the single most important risk factor for dementia, and particularly AD. Other sociodemographic factors have also been identified, including sex, level of education, quality of social networks and activities, physical exercise, smoking and alcohol consumption.

Gender

The vast majority of prevalence data suggest that dementia is more frequent in women than in men. Indeed, various authors have reported a higher prevalence of dementia in women, regardless of the origin of the population studied (Bachman *et al.* 1992; Bowirrat, Friedland and Korczyn 2002; Corso *et al.* 1992; Graves *et al.* 1996; Jorm, Korten and Henderson 1987; Kiyohara *et al.* 1994; Manubens *et al.* 1995; Rocca *et al.* 1991; Wilson *et al.* 2005a; Woo *et al.* 1998; Zhou *et al.* 2006), although a few studies have reported an identical prevalence of dementia across the two sexes (Hebert *et al.* 2001; Liu *et al.* 1995; Pfeffer, Afifi and Chance 1987; Prencipe *et al.* 1996; Skoog *et al.* 1993; Yamada *et al.* 1999).

This result could be explained by different factors. First, the duration of the disease may be longer in women than in men, since they may survive longer: a US study of more than 500 incident cases of AD reported that median survival in men was 4.2 years compared to 5.7 years for women (Larson *et al.* 2004). Another explanation could be a higher frequency of dementia risk factors in women, including hormonal and genetic factors, as well as sociocultural factors such as a low level of education. However, one study which took into account both sex and level of education simultaneously still found an increased incidence of dementia in women (Letenneur *et al.* 1999).

This sex difference has not been observed in all incidence studies, but two meta-analyses (Gao *et al.* 1998; Launer *et al.* 1999) concluded that AD incidence was higher in women. In fact, it seems the sex differences in incidence are also related to age: in the Paquid study, the incidence of both AD and all-cause dementia was found to be higher in men before 80 years, but higher in women after 80 years (Letenneur *et al.* 1999).

Level of education

A low level of education, evaluated either by the number of years of formal education or the highest educational qualification achieved, is often associated with an increased risk of developing AD in many (Fratiglioni *et al.* 1991; Hill *et al.* 1993; Letenneur *et al.* 2000; Ott *et al.* 1995; Stern *et al.* 1994; Sulkava *et al.* 1985) although not all (Beard *et al.* 1992; Cobb *et al.* 1995; O'Connor, Pollitt and Treasure 1991) cohort studies. Several factors could explain this association between education and dementia risk. First, education may increase 'cognitive reserve' which seems to modulate the clinical expression of AD pathology and may delay diagnosis (Stern 2006). People with low levels of education might be involved in less demanding cognitive tasks later on in life, leading to lower brain stimulation and lower cognitive reserve. These individuals might also be more likely to be exposed to toxic substances, which could also be risk factors for dementia, since they are more likely to have rural or manual occupations (Letenneur *et al.* 1999).

There may also be an element of diagnostic bias, since patients with lower levels of education generally have poorer performances on neuropsychological tests, and so are more easily identified and diagnosed in epidemiological studies. People with higher levels of education seem to show better performances in particular on tests of executive function (Le Carret *et al.* 2003), perhaps due to their capacities of cognitive reserve (Letenneur *et al.* 2000; Mortimer and Graves 1993; Satz *et al.* 1993; Stern *et al.* 1992).

Level of education is also an indicator of socioeconomic status, but the relationship between education and dementia seems to be independent of socioeconomic status (Helmer *et al.* 2001; Ravaglia *et al.* 2002; Richards *et al.* 2004) or income (Evans *et al.* 1997; Karp *et al.* 2004).

There have not yet been any 'life-course' studies enabling us to clearly understand the role of social inequalities in cerebral aging. It appears that the education effect plays a role well before the diagnosis of dementia, since in cognitively normal individuals the risk of converting to the stage of mild cognitive impairment (MCI) is greater in those with a lower level of education (Kryscio et al. 2006).

Some studies have found that a high socioeconomic status was associated with a decreased risk of AD (Evans et al. 1997; Letenneur et al. 1999; Stern et al. 1994), but these studies were limited by the fact that socioeconomic status was only measured at the time of disease onset. More recent studies have shown that socioeconomic status during early life can influence cognitive function in later life, but not the risk of AD or cognitive decline (Wilson et al. 2005b).

Lifestyle

SOCIAL NETWORK, SOCIAL ACTIVITIES AND COGNITIVE STIMULATION

Numerous studies have suggested a protective role of strong social networks and social activities on cognitive decline (Barnes et al. 2004; Holtzman et al. 2004; Scarmeas et al. 2001). A review of 15 longitudinal studies in Europe and the US found an overall beneficial effect of strong social networks and social activities, whether or not they are intellectually stimulating, on cognition and the risk of dementia (Fratiglioni et al. 2004).

In a study of elderly people, a protective effect of leisure activities on the incidence of MCI was only found for cognitively stimulating activities. This effect was robust and persisted even after the exclusion of participants who developed dementia during the first two years of follow-up (Verghese et al. 2006).

Marital status could be an indicator of strong social networks, and some studies have shown that it could play a protective role against AD (Fratiglioni et al. 2000; Helmer et al. 1999). Other studies show that leisure activities, such as reading, games, dancing, gardening, DIY and travel, are associated with a lower risk of AD and other dementias (Fabrigoule et al. 1995). In contrast, less cognitively stimulating activities, such as watching television, are thought to be associated with a greater risk of cognitive impairment (Wang et al. 2006). However, it is difficult to exclude the hypothesis that decreased participation in leisure activities during the early stages of the disease could lead to an overestimation of the effect of such factors. Indeed, the majority of studies have been carried out in populations aged 65 or over, but a recent study of 2513 men evaluated the effect of social engagement in both midlife and late life. The authors found that social engagement in midlife alone was not associated with the risk of dementia. This result could be in favour of the hypothesis that levels of late-life social engagement could be modified by the dementing process and may be associated with prodromal dementia (Saczynski *et al.* 2006). Another recent study showed that social network size may modify the relation between AD neuropathology (in particular neurofibrillary tangles) and the level of cognitive function (Bennett *et al.* 2006).

It remains difficult to conceptualize and quantify social activities and networks in epidemiological studies, since beyond the simple existence of these activities it would also seem important to take into account the satisfaction gained from them.

Many studies have demonstrated a relationship between increased participation in cognitive activities in late life and a decreased risk of dementia (Karp *et al.* 2006; Scarmeas *et al.* 2001; Verghese *et al.* 2003; Wang *et al.* 2002), AD (Verghese *et al.* 2003; Wilson *et al.* 2002a, 2002b, 2007), vascular dementia (VaD) (Verghese *et al.* 2003) or cognitive decline or impairment (Bosma *et al.* 2002; Hultsch *et al.* 1999; Verghese *et al.* 2006; Wang *et al.* 2006; Wilson *et al.* 2002b, 2003). One longitudinal study assessing the impact of intellectually demanding work on cognitive performance found a significant interaction between level of intelligence and intellectually demanding work: the positive association between intellectually demanding work and cognitive performance was stronger in individuals with lower intellectual aptitude, suggesting that behaviour may enhance intellectual reserve, even many years after the end of formal education (Potter, Helms and Plassman 2008).

A randomized controlled trial of three types of cognitive training (memory, reasoning and speed of processing) in older adults found that each of three cognitive interventions improved the cognitive ability it targeted and this improvement continued five years after the initiation of the intervention (Willis *et al.* 2006). Furthermore, reasoning training resulted in less functional decline in self-reported instrumental activities of daily living (Willis *et al.* 2006).

PHYSICAL EXERCISE

Numerous longitudinal population-based studies carried out in participants aged 65 years or more have reported an inverse association between regular and sustained physical activities and the presence of cognitive decline (Lytle *et al.* 2004; Van Gelder *et al.* 2004; Weuve *et al.* 2004; Yaffe *et al.* 2001) or dementia, in particular AD (Abbott *et al.* 2004; Larson *et al.* 2006; Podewils *et al.* 2005). The credibility of these results is strengthened by the high methodological quality of these studies (sufficient statistical power, long duration of follow-up, longitudinal analysis). Meta-analyses of prospective longitudinal studies have also concluded that physical activity has a beneficial effect on the risk of cognitive decline (Sofi *et al.* 2011) and dementia (Hamer and Chida 2009).

Only a few relatively small intervention studies have been carried out, and some (Kramer *et al.* 1999; Lautenschlager *et al.* 2008), but not all (Oken *et al.* 2006), have demonstrated beneficial effects of some forms of physical exercise on cognitive outcome measures in elderly populations. However, large-scale intervention studies are required to determine the true effects of standardized physical exercise programmes on cognition.

SMOKING

Initial results suggesting a protective effect of smoking on the development of AD (Graves *et al.* 1991; Lee 1994; Van Duijn *et al.* 1994) are most likely due to selective survival bias (Doll *et al.* 1994; Hernan, Alonso and Logroscino 2008; Riggs 1993), since they have not been confirmed by more recent studies. Indeed, analysis of longitudinal data suggests an increased risk of developing dementia or AD amongst smokers (Brenner *et al.* 1993; Cervilla, Prince and Mann 2000; Hebert *et al.* 1992; Launer *et al.* 1999; Merchant *et al.* 1999; Prince, Cullen and Mann 1994; Yoshitake *et al.* 1995). One study even found a dose-response effect between the level of smoking exposure and the risk of AD (Juan *et al.* 2004), while other studies only found an association in non-apolipoprotein (APOE) ε4 carriers (Ott *et al.* 1998). One large-scale study that followed up 9209 participants for 2.3 years suggested the cumulative smoking exposure, measured by the number of pack-years, may accelerate cognitive decline in individuals without dementia with a dose-response effect (Ott *et al.* 2004).

ALCOHOL

The Paquid study was the first to suggest that alcohol may be protective against dementia (Lemeshow *et al.* 1998). Since then, other studies have also generally shown a protective effect of moderate alcohol, but not necessarily wine, consumption on the risk of dementia (Letenneur, Larrieu and Barberger-Gateau 2004; Peters *et al.* 2008) or cognitive decline (Anstey, Mack and Cherbuin 2009). Various explanations for this association have been proposed, including (i) that moderate alcohol consumption may be associated with an overall 'protective' lifestyle; (ii) that moderate alcohol consumption may decrease cardiovascular risk; (iii) a direct action of alcohol on the acetylcholine metabolism; or (iv) specifically for wine, a protective role of its flavanoid components (Savaskan *et al.* 2003). However, it remains unclear whether the association between alcohol and cognition reflects selection bias in cohort studies commencing in late life, a protective effect of alcohol consumption throughout adulthood, or a specific benefit of alcohol in late life (Anstey et al. 2009).

Nutrition

Aging is associated with a reduction of both micro- and macro-nutrient intakes, as well as with modifications in the absorption and metabolism of nutrients. Studies of the association between nutrition and cognition must take into account the fact that cognitive impairment may bring about modifications in eating behaviours and therefore could be a cause rather than a result of nutritional deficiencies. Longitudinal studies with sufficiently long follow-up periods are therefore required to ensure the temporal relationship between nutritional status and cognition is properly elucidated.

Homocysteine, B-vitamins and folate

There is conflicting evidence from longitudinal observational studies about the association between homocysteine and homocysteine-lowering vitamins and cognition or dementia:

- Many studies have found increased homocysteine levels in older people to be associated with an increased risk of dementia or cognitive decline (Haan et al. 2007; Ravaglia et al. 2005; Seshadri et al. 2002), or increased intake or serum levels of homocysteine-lowering vitamins (vitamins B6, B12 and folate) to be associated with a decreased risk (Clarke et al. 2007; Corrada et al. 2005; Kado et al. 2005; Luchsinger et al. 2007; Morris et al. 2005a; Ravaglia et al. 2005; Tucker et al. 2005; Wang et al. 2001).

- A large number of studies have found no association (Clarke et al. 2007; Corrada et al. 2005; Crystal et al. 1994; Kalmijn et al. 1999; Kang et al. 2006b; Luchsinger et al. 2004, 2007; Mooijaart et al. 2005; Morris et al. 2006; Ravaglia et al. 2005; Teunissen et al. 2003)

- One study (Morris et al. 2005a) even suggested that increased dietary folate intake was associated with increased cognitive decline.

A number of randomized trials have been conducted to determine the effects of folic acid, alone or in combination with other B-vitamins, on cognition, but results have again been inconsistent. A recent Cochrane meta-analysis concluded that there is 'no consistent evidence either way that folic acid, with or without vitamin B12, has a beneficial effect on cognitive function of unselected healthy or cognitively impaired older people' (Malouf and Grimley Evans 2008).

Antioxidants

- In some prospective longitudinal studies, people with higher intakes (either through diet or supplements) of antioxidants, particularly vitamins E and C, have been found to have slower cognitive decline and a lower risk of AD in old age, but other studies have found no association (Gillette-Guyonnet *et al.* 2007).

- There is little evidence of a protective effect of antioxidants on cognition from randomized controlled trials (Yaffe *et al.* 2004), although few trials have been conducted so far.

Ginkgo biloba, which has, amongst other proposed actions, powerful antioxidant properties, has also been tested in randomized trials:

- A 3.5-year trial in 118 elderly persons aged 85 years or older found no significant effect of Ginkgo biloba on cognitive decline overall, but did find a protective effect once compliance was taken into account (Dodge *et al.* 2008).

- The first large-scale trial of Ginkgo biloba for the prevention of dementia found no effect (DeKosky *et al.* 2008) following a median of six years' supplementation in 3069 elderly participants, and the results of the second large-scale prevention trial (Andrieu *et al.* 2008) have not yet been published.

Vitamin D

Vitamin D has recently been suggested as a potentially protective factor against dementia, but only two longitudinal studies have been carried out:

- One found low levels of vitamin D to be associated with substantial cognitive decline in the elderly population studied over a six-year period (Llewellyn *et al.* 2010).

- The other found little evidence of independent associations between lower vitamin D level and incident cognitive decline in a cohort of elderly men (Slinin *et al.* 2010).

Fatty acids and fish consumption

- Several longitudinal studies have suggested that a higher intake of polyunsaturated (PUFA) or monounsaturated (MUFA) fatty acids could be associated with a lower risk of dementia or cognitive impairment (Laitinen *et al.* 2006; Morris *et al.* 2003a; Solfrizzi *et al.* 2006a, 2006b).

- One study found no association between low intakes of MUFA, n-3 PUFA or n-6 PUFA and dementia (Engelhart *et al.* 2002).

- High plasma phosphatidycholine docosahexaenoic acid (DHA; an omega-3 fatty acid found in cold-water fatty fish and fish oil supplements) was also associated with a decreased risk of dementia, but not AD, in one study (Schaefer *et al.* 2006) and with less cognitive decline in two other studies (Beydoun *et al.* 2007; Dullemeijer *et al.* 2007).

- Other studies have found higher fish consumption to be associated with a decreased risk of dementia or cognitive decline (Barberger-Gateau *et al.* 2002, 2007; Huang *et al.* 2005; Kalmijn *et al.* 1997; Morris *et al.* 2003b, 2005b; Van Gelder *et al.* 2007).

- One randomized controlled trial assessed the effects of two-year supplementation with n-3 long-chain polyunsaturated fatty acid and found no effect on cognitive function in 867 cognitive healthy adults aged 70–79 years (Dangour *et al.* 2010).

Dietary patterns

- The conflicting results arising from studies of individual nutrients could reflect the fact that one nutrient alone may not be enough to affect cognition or risk of dementia, and it could be that a balanced combination of several nutrients may be required for prevention of cognitive decline or dementia (Gillette-Guyonnet *et al.* 2007).

- There have been few studies of dietary patterns on the risk of dementia, but one longitudinal observational study suggested that a diverse diet may reduce the risk of dementia (Barberger-Gateau *et al.* 2007) and a second found a decreased risk of AD in participants following a Mediterranean-style diet (Scarmeas *et al.* 2006).

Obesity and body composition

Three meta-analyses (Anstey *et al.* 2011; Beydoun, Beydoun and Wang 2008; Gorospe and Dave 2007) concluded that:

- Underweight body mass index (BMI), overweight BMI and obese BMI in midlife were all associated with an increased risk of dementia in late life compared with normal midlife BMI.

- There may be a U-shaped relationship, with highest risks for underweight and obese BMI.

- Results regarding the association between late-life BMI and dementia risk were unclear, although the same U-shaped relationship could potentially exist.

Vascular risk factors

Hypertension

The relation between blood pressure, cognitive function and dementia has been assessed in numerous epidemiological studies. A comprehensive review of observational population-based studies published in 2005 (Qiu, Winblad and Fratiglioni 2005), which took into account the effects of age on the relationship between blood pressure and cognition, concluded that high blood pressure in midlife is a risk factor for cognitive impairment and dementia (including AD) in late life. Results were inconsistent for the effects of late-life blood pressure, but there was a suggestion that low blood pressure in late life may be associated with poorer cognition. A recent population-based longitudinal study found that low diastolic blood pressure predicted the risk of dementia among very old people, and suggested that blood pressure exhibits a substantial decline over approximately three years before the clinical onset of the dementia syndrome (Qiu, Winblad and Fratiglioni 2009). Low blood pressure may be related to the actual dementing process itself rather than being a true risk factor.

There is also some observational evidence to suggest that antihypertensive treatment may have some beneficial effects against cognitive decline and dementia in elderly people (Qiu et al. 2005). However, a recent Cochrane meta-analysis (McGuinness et al. 2009b), including four randomized controlled trials involving 15,936 hypertensive participants, concluded that there was no convincing evidence that blood pressure lowering in late life can prevent dementia or cognitive impairment in hypertensive patients without prior cerebrovascular disease.

Diabetes

A literature review of 14 longitudinal studies (Biessels et al. 2006) concluded that there is convincing evidence of an increased risk of dementia (AD, vascular dementia and mixed dementia) in people with diabetes. Two other reviews (Allen, Frier and Strachan 2004; Cukierman, Gerstein and Williamson 2005) studied the relationship between diabetes and cognitive decline and concluded that, compared to people without diabetes, people with diabetes have a 1.5-fold greater risk of cognitive decline. However, there are few details on the modulating and mediating effects of glycemic control, other vascular risk factors and micro vascular complications.

The prevention or treatment of diabetes could therefore potentially be used to prevent dementia (Luchsinger 2010), although no results are yet available from randomized controlled trials. The effects of long-term glycemic control on cognitive decline and structural brain changes in patients with type 2 diabetes were measured in the ACCORD-MIND study (Williamson et al. 2007), a sub-study of the ACCORD trial, and cognitive testing has now also been added (Luchsinger 2010) to the Finnish Diabetes Prevention Study (Tuomilehto et al. 2001) and the Diabetes Prevention Program Outcomes Study (Knowler et al. 2009) which demonstrated the efficacy of lifestyle interventions on diabetes prevention.

Cholesterol

Several observational studies have found an association between high serum cholesterol levels and the risk of dementia or AD. However, as with hypertension, it appears that it is cholesterol levels during midlife that have the most important effect on late-life cognition and risk of dementia (Anstey, Lipnicki and Low 2008).

Initial observational studies (including cross-sectional and case-control studies) suggested that the use of statins (cholesterol-lowering drugs) was associated with a decreased risk of dementia (Jick et al. 2000; Rockwood et al. 2002) or AD (Wolozin et al. 2000) or lower odds of cognitive impairment (Yaffe et al. 2002). Also, one study suggested an association between antecedent statin use and neurofibrillary tangle burden at autopsy (Li et al. 2007). However, three recent large prospective studies found no association between statin use and the risk of dementia or AD (Li et al. 2004; Rea et al. 2005; Zandi et al. 2005).

Furthermore, large randomized controlled trials have not found any benefit of statins for the prevention of dementia or preservation of cognition (McGuinness et al. 2009a).

Pharmacological treatments

Hormone replacement therapy

Following suggestions of a protective effect of oestrogen or hormone replacement therapy (HRT) on the risk of dementia or cognitive function in observational studies, a number of randomized controlled trials have been conducted. The most recent Cochrane meta-analysis (2008) concluded that there is good evidence that both oestrogen replacement therapy and HRT do not prevent cognitive decline in older postmenopausal women when given as short-term or longer-term (up to five years) therapy (Lethaby et al. 2008).

The Women's Health Initiative Memory Study (WHIMS), a randomized controlled trial conducted in nearly 7500 community-dwelling postmenopausal women, found that oestrogen plus progestin therapy increased the risk for probable dementia (Shumaker *et al.* 2003) and that oestrogen therapy alone did not reduce dementia or MCI incidence, and increased the risk for both endpoints combined (Shumaker *et al.* 2004).

Non-steroidal anti-inflammatory drugs

An initial meta-analysis (Etminan, Gill and Samii 2003) and systematic review (Szekely *et al.* 2004) suggested that non-steroidal anti-inflammatory drugs (NSAIDs) had a protective effect on the risk of AD. However, a more recent meta-analysis concluded that most of the reported beneficial effects of NSAIDs in observational studies could well be the result of bias (de Craen *et al.* 2005). Moreover, two RCTs have found no effects of NSAIDs (Lyketsos *et al.* 2007) or aspirin (Kang *et al.* 2007) on dementia or cognitive decline. In the ADAPT study (Lyketsos *et al.* 2007), specifically designed as a dementia primary prevention trial, but prematurely terminated due to safety concerns, celecoxib and naproxen showed trends for increased risks of AD compared to placebo in 2528 participants aged 70 years and older. The WHS cognitive cohort (Kang *et al.* 2007) involved 6377 women aged over 65 treated with low-dose aspirin or placebo for 9.6 years on average. Active treatment had no effect on cognitive performance or decline at either cognitive assessment.

Discrepancies between observational and interventional studies

Although some risk factors for dementia such as age, sex and socioeconomic status are essentially non-modifiable, many of the risk or protective factors identified in epidemiological research could be modified through intervention. However, formal guidelines concerning the use of pharmacological, nutritional or other interventions for the prevention of dementia can only be put into place for routine medical practice if their efficacy is proven in randomized controlled trials. As highlighted earlier, some trials have now been carried out to test the efficacy of interventions targeting modifiable risk factors on the risk of dementia or the preservation of cognitive function. However, despite suggested positive effects in observational studies, so far results have been disappointing in randomized trials, in particular for the few trials that assessed dementia incidence as a primary endpoint (DeKosky *et al.* 2008; Lyketsos *et al.* 2007; Shumaker *et al.* 2003, 2004).

Hormone replacement therapy is a classic example of a factor that appeared to be protective against dementia in observational studies, but which raised numerous safety concerns, in particular the possibility of it actually increasing the risk of dementia, in randomized controlled trials (Shumaker *et al.* 2003, 2004). Safety concerns, although unrelated to dementia risk, have also led to the suspension of prevention trials testing NSAIDs (Lyketsos *et al.* 2007) or diabetes control methods (Williamson *et al.* 2007). The safety of interventions tested in prevention trials is of vital importance, given that they are tested in essentially healthy individuals, many of whom may not actually go on to develop dementia or AD.

An analysis of the observational and interventional studies carried out in the field of dementia prevention has suggested a number of methodological reasons that could explain the discrepancies between results from observational and interventional studies (Coley *et al.* 2008).

A first explanation for these differing results can be focused on the methodology of the observational studies. By design, observational studies are more prone to bias and more confounding than randomized controlled trials, which are generally considered the 'gold standard' of epidemiological research (McKee *et al.* 1999). A whole range of potential biases can invalidate the results of observational studies (Delgado-Rodriguez and Llorca 2004). Although the previous section focused on prospective longitudinal studies in order to ensure that temporal relationships were properly accounted for, other forms of bias may have affected the observational studies; for example: measurement bias, confounding, healthy user bias, protopathic bias and attrition bias.

Aside from the problems of bias and confounding in observational studies, a number of other methodological explanations could explain the inconsistencies in results between observational and experimental studies.

1. Study population

The people who agree to participate in randomized dementia prevention trials are a highly selected population of individuals who probably differ from those who do not take part in terms of education, health behaviours and general lifestyle (Green and DeKosky 2006). Indeed, many prevention trials have had lower than expected dementia incidence rates or less cognitive decline than expected, perhaps because participants are 'too healthy'. This makes it more difficult to detect treatment effects because of a lack of statistical power. Also, those enrolled in prevention trials are probably those who are least susceptible to the intervention, since they may already have a relatively healthy lifestyle in terms of diet, exercise, social contacts, etc., or they may already be receiving nutritional fortification through public health measures.

2. Design of the intervention

There may also be major differences between the nature of the interventions used in prevention trials, and the nature of the risk/protective factors studied in observational studies. For example, vitamin E exists in several different forms, more than one of which may be required for a protective effect on cognition (Morris *et al.* 2005c). In the Women's Health Study, a supplement containing only the α-tocopherol form was used, and no effect was observed on cognition (Kang *et al.* 2006a), but the observational studies assessing vitamin E as a protective factor may have studied other forms of this vitamin. The dose of treatments tested in randomized trials is also an important consideration.

3. Window of exposure

Another potential difference between observational and interventional studies is the 'window of exposure'; that is, the time of life at which individuals are exposed to the intervention. This has been particularly discussed in the domain of HRT: it has been suggested that treatment needs to be started around the immediate post-menopausal period for a beneficial effect (Henderson 2006; Maki 2006), but the participants enrolled in prevention trials were perhaps too old (65 years and older at baseline) to benefit from HRT. Likewise, some observational evidence suggests that NSAID use, hypertension or elevated cholesterol in midlife rather than late life may be beneficial against dementia or cognitive decline (Qiu *et al.* 2005; t' Veld *et al.* 2001), but prevention trials focusing on these factors have so far only been carried out in late life.

4. Duration of intervention and follow-up

Another difference between observational and intervention studies was the duration of follow-up. For example, in studies in the domain of nutrition, the duration of follow-up in the longitudinal studies was generally three years or more, but only two randomized controlled trials (Durga *et al.* 2007; Kang *et al.* 2006a) were of similar length.

5. Outcome measures

The outcome measures used in observational and interventional studies could also explain some of the conflicting results. For example, all of the randomized trials testing a nutritional supplement assessed the effects of the intervention on cognitive decline, but many observational studies assessed the association between nutrients and dementia incidence rather than cognitive decline. It has not yet been proven that cognitive decline is a surrogate marker for the onset of dementia, and so the two endpoints cannot be used interchangeably. Furthermore, numerous cognitive tests exist which can target either global cognitive function, or individual cognitive domains, such as episodic memory or executive function, and so a positive effect may be observed with certain measures but not others.

6. Insufficient statistical power

Some of the smaller prevention trials, in particular those testing HRT (Almeida *et al.* 2006; Binder *et al.* 2001; Polo-Kantola *et al.* 1998; Viscoli *et al.* 2005) or Ginkgo biloba (Carlson *et al.* 2007; Dodge *et al.* 2008; Wesnes *et al.* 2000), have not reported sample size calculations, and so it is not possible to determine whether or not they were sufficiently powered to be able to detect treatment effects. However, given the small numbers of participants and short length of follow-up, many were likely to be statistically underpowered.

7. Attrition bias

Attrition (dropout) may also affect the detection of treatment effects in randomized controlled trials, either through decreasing statistical power or through bias. For example, in the SHEP study, which found no effect of antihypertensive treatment on cognitive decline or dementia, sensitivity analyses suggested that differential dropout may have obscured potential treatment effects (Di Bari *et al.* 2001).

8. The need for multidomain interventions

All of the prevention trials carried out so far have targeted only one type of risk factor, but given the multifactorial nature of dementia, in particular AD, interventions acting on only one individual risk factor may not be enough. Indeed, an observational study (Scarmeas *et al.* 2009) found that adherence to a Mediterranean-type diet and participating in physical activity were independently associated with a decreased risk of developing AD, and that individuals with both the highest dietary adherence and the highest levels of physical activity had the lowest risk of developing AD.

The first randomized trials testing multidomain interventions for the prevention of cognitive decline or dementia are now under way, and include the MAPT (Gillette-Guyonnet *et al.* 2009), FINGER (Kivipelto undated) and PreDIVA (Richard *et al.* 2009) studies.

Conclusion

Without intervention, the global burden of dementia is set to increase dramatically in the coming years in both developed and developing countries. Epidemiological research has identified numerous candidates for modifiable risk factors, but interventions focused on these factors have so far been unsuccessful when tested in randomized trials. While the interventions tested may truly have been ineffective, methodological problems could also explain some of the failed trials. Further prevention trials are therefore merited, and particular attention should be paid to the methodology of such trials, aiming to ensure that they bring about conditions similar to those that have been suggested as protective in observational studies.

Even interventions with fairly modest effects could have a strong influence on the future burden of dementia. For example, in AD it has been suggested that an intervention able to delay disease onset and progression by just one year would bring about a reduction of more than 9 million cases of the disease by 2050, and it is thought that much of this decline in prevalence would be attributable to decreases in persons needing a high level of care (Brookmeyer et al. 2007).

Without clear evidence from randomized trials, no formal guidelines can be put into place for routine medical practice concerning the prevention of cognitive decline or dementia. In particular, treatment of vascular risk factors, and the use of NSAIDs and HRT, cannot be recommended for this purpose at the current time. However, certain lifestyle changes can be suggested concerning, for example, diet, exercise and social engagement, even without a lack of definitive evidence of their effects on dementia incidence. Such lifestyle changes are unlikely to have any harmful effects and could well improve quality of life and overall health, in addition to their potentially protective effects against dementia.

Glossary of epidemiological study terms

Case-control study A type of *observational* study in which patients who have developed a disease (or other outcome of interest) are identified and their past exposure to suspected aetiological factors is compared with that of controls or referents who do not have the disease. The main disadvantages are the retrospective nature of exposure assessment (increasing the risk of bias) and the difficulty in defining controls.

Cohort study Study comparing the occurrence of a disease or other outcome of interest (e.g. cognitive decline) in groups of individuals classed as either exposed or unexposed to a given risk or protective factor. Cohort studies are *observational* studies that may be *prospective* or *retrospective*.

Cross-sectional study A type of *observational* study measuring the prevalence of health outcomes or determinants of health, or both, in a group of individuals at a single point in time (or over a short period). Exposures and outcomes of interest are measured simultaneously, meaning that it is impossible to draw conclusions regarding temporal relationships.

Delphi consensus study A group of experts are asked to give their opinion or estimate concerning a given question, based on their own qualitative assessment of existing evidence. Experts' estimates are aggregated and fed back anonymously to all participants, who then review their initial responses in view of group-wide choices. The group does not need to meet to reach a decision (the process can be done by telephone, email, fax, etc.).

Experimental study Study in which the investigator determines who is exposed and who is unexposed to a factor or intervention or interest.

Longitudinal study Study in which participants are followed over time with continuous or repeated monitoring of risk factors or health outcomes, or both.

Meta-analysis Systematic, organized and structured evaluation of a problem of interest. Data from a set of comparable studies on a given topic are combined and analysed to give a quantitative summary of the included studies. All eligible studies relevant to the question of interest must be identified using a systematic search strategy using predetermined criteria. The methodology of the identified studies is critically appraised in order to determine if it is of sufficient quality to be included in the meta-analysis.

Observational study Study drawing inferences about the possible effect of a treatment or other exposure of interest on a given outcome, where the assignment of subjects to the 'exposed' and 'unexposed' groups is outside the control of the investigator. The main disadvantage of this type of study is that the groups may differ for characteristics other than the exposure of interest, which can result in biased results.

Pooled study A combined analysis of two or more studies involving aggregation of the data from the individual studies.

Population-based study Study in which a sample, or even the entirety, of a defined population is included. The main advantage of this type of study is its external validity, i.e. the applicability of its results to a defined population.

Prospective study Study in which exposure and covariate measurements are made before cases of illness (or other outcomes of interest) occur.

Randomized controlled trial Study in which participants are allocated at random to receive one of several clinical interventions (often drug treatments, but may also include screening programmes, lifestyle modifications, surgical procedures, etc.). The effects of the interventions are examined on the occurrence of a disease or other outcome of interest (e.g. death, cognitive decline). The main advantage of this type of study is that the act of randomizing patients to receive or not receive the intervention ensures that, on average, all other possible prognostic factors (both known and unknown) are equal between the two groups. Thus, any significant differences between groups in the outcome event can be attributed to the intervention. When possible, randomized controlled trials should be 'double-blind', meaning that neither the patient nor the investigator knows which treatment the patient has received.

Retrospective study Study in which exposure and covariate measurements are made after the outcome of interest has already occurred.

Systematic review Literature review aiming to identify, critically appraise and synthesize all relevant studies of a specific topic. *Meta-analysis* may be, but is not necessarily, used as part of this process.

References

Abbott, R.D., White, L.R., Ross, G.W., Masaki, K.H., Curb, J.D. and Petrovitch, H. (2004) 'Walking and dementia in physically capable elderly men.' *Journal of the American Medical Association 292*, 12, 1447–1453.

Allen, K.V., Frier, B.M. and Strachan, M.W. (2004) 'The relationship between type 2 diabetes and cognitive dysfunction: longitudinal studies and their methodological limitations.' *European Journal of Pharmacology 490*, 169–75.

Almeida, O., Lautenschlager, N.T., Vasikaran, S., Leedman, P. *et al.* (2006) 'A 20-week randomized controlled trial of estradiol replacement therapy for women aged 70 years and older: effect on mood, cognition and quality of life.' *Neurobiology of Aging 27*, 141–9.

Alzheimer's Disease International (2010) *World Alzheimer's Report.* London: Alzheimer's Disease International.

Andrieu, S., Ousset, P.J., Coley, N., Ouzid, M., Mathiex-Fortunet, H. and Vellas, B. (2008) 'GuidAge study: a 5-year double blind, randomised trial of EGb 761 for the prevention of Alzheimer's disease in elderly subjects with memory complaints. i. Rationale, design and baseline data.' *Current Alzheimer Research 5*, 406–15.

Anstey, K.J., Cherbuin, N., Budge, M. and Young, J. (2011) 'Body mass index in midlife and late-life as a risk factor for dementia: a meta-analysis of prospective studies.' *Obesity Reviews 12*, e426–37.

Anstey, K.J., Lipnicki, D.M. and Low, L.F. (2008) 'Cholesterol as a risk factor for dementia and cognitive decline: a systematic review of prospective studies with meta-analysis.' *American Journal of Geriatric Psychiatry 16*, 343–54.

Anstey, K.J., Mack, H.A. and Cherbuin, N. (2009) 'Alcohol consumption as a risk factor for dementia and cognitive decline: meta-analysis of prospective studies.' *American Journal of Geriatric Psychiatry 17*, 542–55.

Bachman, D.L., Wolf, P.A., Linn, R., Knoefel, J.E. *et al.* (1992) 'Prevalence of dementia and probable senile dementia of the Alzheimer type in the Framingham Study.' *Neurology 42*, 115–19.

Barberger-Gateau, P., Letenneur, L., Deschamps, V., Peres, K. *et al.* (2002) 'Fish, meat, and risk of dementia: cohort study.' *British Medical Journal 325*, 932–3.

Barberger-Gateau, P., Raffaitin, C., Letenneur, L., Berr, C. *et al.* (2007) 'Dietary patterns and risk of dementia: the Three-City cohort study.' *Neurology 69*, 1921–30.

Barnes, L.L., Mendes De Leon, C.F., Wilson, N.R.S., Bienias, J.L. and Evans, D.A. (2004) 'Social resources and cognitive decline in a population of older African Americans and whites.' *Neurology 63*, 2322–6.

Beard, C.M., Kokmen, E., Offord, K.P. and Kurland, L.T. (1992) 'Lack of association between Alzheimer's disease and education, occupation, marital status, or living arrangement.' *Neurology 42*, 2063–8.

Bennett, D.A., Schneider, J.A., Tang, Y., Arnold, S.E. and Wilson, R.S. (2006) 'The effect of social networks on the relation between Alzheimer's disease pathology and level of cognitive function in old people: a longitudinal cohort study.' *Lancet Neurology 5*, 406–12.

Beydoun, M.A., Beydoun, H.A. and Wang, Y. (2008) 'Obesity and central obesity as risk factors for incident dementia and its subtypes: a systematic review and meta-analysis.' *Obesity Reviews 9*, 204–18.

Beydoun, M.A., Kaufman, J.S., Satia, J.A., Rosamond, W. and Folsom, A.R. (2007) 'Plasma n-3 fatty acids and the risk of cognitive decline in older adults: the Atherosclerosis Risk in Communities Study.' *American Journal of Clinical Nutrition 85*, 1103–11.

Biessels, G.J., Staekenborg, S., Brunner, E., Brayne, C. and Scheltens, P.C. (2006) 'Risk of dementia in diabetes mellitus: a systematic review.' *Lancet Neurology 5*, 64–74.

Binder, E.F., Schechtman, K.B., Birge, S., Williams, D.B. and Kohrt, W.M. (2001) 'Effects of hormone replacement therapy on cognitive performance in elderly women.' *Maturitas 38*, 137–46.

Bosma, H., Van Boxtel, M.P., Ponds, R.W., Jelicic, M. *et al.* (2002) 'Engaged lifestyle and cognitive function in middle and old-aged, non-demented persons: a reciprocal association?' *Zeitschrift für Gerontologie und Geriatrie 35*, 575–81.

Bowirrat, A., Friedland, R.P. and Korczyn, A.D. (2002) 'Vascular dementia among elderly Arabs in Wadi Ara.' *Journal of the Neurological Sciences 203/204*, 73–6.

Brenner, D.E., Kukull, W.A., Van Belle, G., Bowen, J.D. *et al.* (1993) 'Relationship between cigarette smoking and Alzheimer's disease in a population-based case-control study.' *Neurology 43*, 293–300.

Brookmeyer, R., Johnson, E., Ziegler-Graham, K. and Arrighi, H.M. (2007) 'Forecasting the global burden of Alzheimer's disease.' *Alzheimers Dement 3*, 186–91.

Carlson, J.J., Farquahar, J.W., Dinucci, E., Ausserer, L. *et al.* (2007) 'Safety and efficacy of a Ginkgo biloba-containing dietary supplement on cognitive function, quality of life, and platelet function in healthy, cognitively intact older adults.' *Journal of the American Dietetic Association 107*, 422–32.

Cervilla, J.A., Prince, M. and Mann, A. (2000) 'Smoking, drinking, and incident cognitive impairment: a cohort community based study included in the Gospel Oak project.' *Journal of Neurology, Neurosurgery and Psychiatry 68*, 622–6.

Clarke, R., Birks, J., Nexo, E., Ueland, P.M. *et al.* (2007) 'Low vitamin B-12 status and risk of cognitive decline in older adults.' *American Journal of Clinical Nutrition 86*, 1384–91.

Cobb, J., Wolf, P.A., Au, R., White, R. and D'Agostino, R.B. (1995) 'The effect of education on the incidence of dementia and Alzheimer's disease in the Framingham Study.' *Neurology 45*, 1707–12.

Coley, N., Andrieu, S., Gardette, V., Gillette-Guyonnet, S. *et al.* (2008) 'Dementia prevention: methodological explanations for inconsistent results.' *Epidemiologic Reviews 30*, 35–66.

Corrada, M., Kawas, C., Hallfrisch, J., Muller, D. and Brookmeyer, R. (2005) 'Reduced risk of Alzheimer's disease with high folate intake: the Baltimore longitudinal study of aging.' *Alzheimer's and Dementia: The Journal of the Alzheimer's Association 1*, 11–18.

Corso, E.A., Campo, G., Triglio, A., Napoli, A. *et al.* (1992) 'Prevalence of moderate and severe Alzheimer dementia and multi-infarct dementia in the population of southeastern Sicily.' *Italian Journal of Neurological Sciences 13*, 215–19.

Crystal, H.A., Ortof, E., Frishman, W.H., Gruber, A. *et al.* (1994) 'Serum vitamin B12 levels and incidence of dementia in a healthy elderly population: a report from the Bronx Longitudinal Aging Study.' *Journal of the American Geriatrics Society 42*, 933–6.

Cukierman, T., Gerstein, H.C. and Williamson, J.D.C. (2005) 'Cognitive decline and dementia in diabetes – systematic overview of prospective observational studies.' *Diabetologia 48*, 2460–9.

Dangour, A.D., Allen, E., Elbourne, D., Fasey, N. *et al.* (2010) 'Effect of 2-y n-3 long-chain polyunsaturated fatty acid supplementation on cognitive function in older people: A randomized, double-blind, controlled trial.' *American Journal of Clinical Nutrition 91*, 1725–32.

de Craen, A.J., Gussekloo, J., Vrijsen, B. and Westendorp, R.G. (2005) 'Meta-analysis of nonsteroidal anti-inflammatory drug use and risk of dementia.' *American Journal of Epidemiology 161*, 114–20.

DeKosky, S.T., Williamson, J.D., Fitzpatrick, A.L., Kronmal, R.A. *et al.* (2008) 'Ginkgo biloba for prevention of dementia: a randomized controlled trial.' *Journal of the American Medical Association 300*, 2253–62.

Delgado-Rodriguez, M. and Llorca, J. (2004) 'Bias.' *Journal of Epidemiology and Community Health 58*, 635–41.

Di Bari, M., Pahor, M., Franse, L.V., Shorr, R.I. *et al.* (2001) 'Dementia and disability outcomes in large hypertension trials: lessons learned from the systolic hypertension in the elderly program (SHEP) trial.' *American Journal of Epidemiology 153*, 72–8.

Dodge, H.H., Zitzelberger, T., Oken, B.S., Howieson, D. and Kaye, J. (2008) 'A randomized placebo-controlled trial of Ginkgo biloba for the prevention of cognitive decline.' *Neurology 70*, 1809–17.

Doll, R., Peto, R., Wheatley, K., Gray, R. and Sutherland, I. (1994) 'Mortality in relation to smoking: 40 years' observations on male British doctors.' *British Medical Journal 309*, 901–11.

Dullemeijer, C., Durga, J., Brouwer, I.A., Van De Rest, O. *et al.* (2007) 'n-3 fatty-acid proportions in plasma and cognitive performance in older adults.' *American Journal of Clinical Nutrition 86*, 1479–85.

Durga, J., Van Boxtel, M.P., Schouten, E.G., Kok, F.J. *et al.* (2007) 'Effect of 3-year folic acid supplementation on cognitive function in older adults in the FACIT trial: a randomised, double blind, controlled trial.' *Lancet 369*, 208–16.

Engelhart, M.J., Geerlings, M.I., Ruitenberg, A., Van Swieten, J.C. *et al.* (2002) 'Diet and risk of dementia: does fat matter? The Rotterdam Study.' *Neurology 59*, 1915–21.

Etminan, M., Gill, S. and Samii, A. (2003) 'Effect of non-steroidal anti-inflammatory drugs on risk of Alzheimer's disease: systematic review and meta-analysis of observational studies.' *British Medical Journal 327*, 128.

Evans, D.A., Hebert, L.E., Beckett, L.A., Scherr, P.A. *et al.* (1997) 'Education and other measures of socioeconomic status and risk of incident Alzheimer disease in a defined population of older persons.' *Archives of Neurology 54*, 1399–405.

Fabrigoule, C., Letenneur, L., Dartigues, J.F., Zarrouk, M. *et al.* (1995) 'Social and leisure activities and risk of dementia: a prospective longitudinal study.' *Journal of the American Geriatrics Society 43*, 485–90.

Ferri, C.P., Prince, M., Brayne, C., Brodaty, H. *et al.* (2005) 'Global prevalence of dementia: a Delphi consensus study.' *Lancet 366*, 2112–17.

Fratiglioni, L., Grut, M., Forsell, Y., Viitanen, M. *et al.* (1991) 'Prevalence of Alzheimer's disease and other dementias in an elderly urban population: relationship with age, sex, and education.' *Neurology 41*, 1886–92.

Fratiglioni, L., Launer, L.J., Andersen, K., Breteler, M.M. *et al.* (2000) 'Incidence of dementia and major subtypes in Europe: a collaborative study of population-based cohorts.' Neurologic Diseases in the Elderly Research Group. *Neurology 54*, S10–15.

Fratiglioni, L., Paillard-Borg, S. and Winblad, B. (2004) 'An active and socially integrated lifestyle in late life might protect against dementia.' *Lancet Neurology 3*, 343–53.

Gao, S., Hendrie, H.C., Hall, K.S. and Hui, S. (1998) 'The relationships between age, sex, and the incidence of dementia and Alzheimer disease: a meta-analysis.' *Archives of General Psychiatry 55*, 809–15.

Gillette-Guyonnet, S., Aandrieu, S., Dantoine, T., Dartigues, J.F. *et al.* (2009) 'Commentary on "A roadmap for the prevention of dementia II. Leon Thal Symposium (2008)". The Multidomain Alzheimer Preventive Trial (MAPT): a new approach to the prevention of Alzheimer's disease.' *Alzheimers Dement 5*, 114–21.

Gillette-Guyonnet, S., Abellan Van Kan, G., Andrieu, S., Barberger-Gateau, P. *et al.* (2007) 'IANA task force on nutrition and cognitive decline with aging.' *Journal of Nutrition Health and Aging 11*, 132–52.

Gorospe, E.C. and Dave, J.K. (2007) 'The risk of dementia with increased body mass index.' *Age and Ageing 36*, 23–9.

Graves, A.B., Larson, E.B., Edland, S.D., Bowen, J.D. *et al.* (1996) 'Prevalence of dementia and its subtypes in the Japanese American population of King County, Washington state: the Kame Project.' *American Journal of Epidemiology 144*, 760–71.

Graves, A.B., Van Duijn, C.M., Chandra, V., Fratiglioni, L. *et al.* (1991) 'Alcohol and tobacco consumption as risk factors for Alzheimer's disease: a collaborative re-analysis of case-control studies. EURODEM Risk Factors Research Group.' *International Journal of Epidemiology 20*, Suppl 2, S48–57.

Green, R.C. and DeKosky, S.T. (2006) 'Primary prevention trials in Alzheimer disease.' *Neurology 67*, S2–5.

Haan, M.N., Miller, J.W., Aiello, A.E., Whitmer, R.A. *et al.* (2007) 'Homocysteine, B vitamins, and the incidence of dementia and cognitive impairment: results from the Sacramento Area Latino Study on Aging.' *American Journal of Clinical Nutrition 85*, 511–17.

Hamer, M. and Chida, Y. (2009) 'Physical activity and risk of neurodegenerative disease: a systematic review of prospective evidence.' *Psychological Medicine 39*, 3–11.

Hebert, L.E., Scherr, P.A., Beckett, L.A., Funkenstien, H.H. *et al.* (1992) 'Relation of smoking and alcohol consumption to incident Alzheimer's disease.' *American Journal of Epidemiology 135*, 347–55.

Hebert, L.E., Scherr, P.A., McCann, J.J., Bechett, L.A. and Evans, D.A. (2001) 'Is the risk of developing Alzheimer's disease greater for women than for men?' *American Journal of Epidemiology 153*, 132–6.

Helmer, C., Damon, D., Letenneur, L., Fabrigoule, C. *et al.* (1999) 'Marital status and risk of Alzheimer's disease: a French population-based cohort study.' *Neurology 53*, 1953–8.

Helmer, C., Letenneur, L., Rouch, I., Richard-Harston, S. *et al.* (2001) 'Occupation during life and risk of dementia in French elderly community residents.' *Journal of Neurology, Neurosurgery and Psychiatry 71*, 303–9.

Henderson, V.W. (2006) 'Estrogen-containing hormone therapy and Alzheimer's disease risk: understanding discrepant inferences from observational and experimental research.' *Neuroscience 138*, 1031–9.

Hernan, M.A., Alonso, A. and Logroscino, G. (2008) 'Cigarette smoking and dementia: Potential selection bias in the elderly.' *Epidemiology 19*, 448–50.

Hill, L.R., Klauber, M.R., Salmon, D.P., Yu, E.S. *et al.* (1993) 'Functional status, education, and the diagnosis of dementia in the Shanghai survey.' *Neurology 43*, 138–45.

Holtzman, R.E., Rebok, G.W., Saczynski, J.S., Kouzis, A.C. *et al.* (2004) 'Social network characteristics and cognition in middle-aged and older adults.' *The Journals of Gerontology Series B: Psychological Sciences and Social Sciences 59*, P278–84.

Huang, T.L., Zandi, P.P., Tucker, K.L., Fitzpatrick, A.L. *et al.* (2005) 'Benefits of fatty fish on dementia risk are stronger for those without APOE epsilon4.' *Neurology 65*, 1409–14.

Hultsch, D.F., Hertzog, C., Small, B.J. and Dixon, R.A. (1999) 'Use it or lose it: engaged lifestyle as a buffer of cognitive decline in aging?' *Psychology and Aging 14*, 245–63.

Jick, H., Zornberg, G.L., Jick, S.S., Seshadri, S. and Drachman, D.A. (2000) 'Statins and the risk of dementia.' *Lancet 356*, 1627–31.

Jorm, A.F., Korten, A.E. and Henderson, A.S. (1987) 'The prevalence of dementia: a quantitative integration of the literature.' *Acta Psychiatrica Scandinavica 76*, 465–79.

Juan, D., Zhou, D.H., Li, J., Wang, J.Y., Gao, C. and Chen, M. (2004) 'A two-year follow-up study of cigarette smoking and risk of dementia.' *European Journal of Neurology 11*, 277–82.

Kado, D.M., Karlamangla, A.S., Huang, M.H., Troen, A. *et al.* (2005) 'Homocysteine versus the vitamins folate, B6, and B12 as predictors of cognitive function and decline in older high-functioning adults: MacArthur Studies of Successful Aging.' *American Journal of Medicine 118*, 161–7.

Kalmijn, S., Launer, L.J., Lindemans, J., Bots, M.L. *et al.* (1999) 'Total homocysteine and cognitive decline in a community-based sample of elderly subjects: the Rotterdam Study.' *American Journal of Epidemiology 150*, 283–9.

Kalmijn, S., Launer, L.J., Ott, A., Witteman, J.C. *et al.* (1997) 'Dietary fat intake and the risk of incident dementia in the Rotterdam Study.' *Annals of Neurology 42*, 776–82.

Kang, J.H., Cook, N., Manson, J., Buring, J.E. and Grodstein, F. (2006a) 'A randomized trial of vitamin E supplementation and cognitive function in women.' *Archives of Internal Medicine 166*, 2462–8.

Kang, J.H., Irizarry, M.C. and Grodstein, F. (2006b) 'Prospective study of plasma folate, vitamin B12, and cognitive function and decline.' *Epidemiology 17*, 650–7.

Kang, J.H., Cook, N., Manson, J., Buring, J.E. and Grodstein, F. (2007) 'Low dose aspirin and cognitive function in the women's health study cognitive cohort.' *British Medical Journal 334*, 987.

Karp, A., Kareholt, I., Qiu, C., Bellander, T. *et al.* (2004) 'Relation of education and occupation-based socioeconomic status to incident Alzheimer's disease.' *American Journal of Epidemiology 159*, 175–83.

Karp, A., Paillard-Borg, S., Wang, H.X., Silverstein, M. *et al.* (2006) 'Mental, physical and social components in leisure activities equally contribute to decrease dementia risk.' *Dementia and Geriatric Cognitive Disorders 21*, 65–73.

Kivipelto, M. (principal investigator) (undated) *Finnish Intervention Geriatric Study to Prevent Cognitive Impairment and Disability* (FINGER). Not published; listed at http://clinicaltrials.gov/ct/show/NCT01041989

Kiyohara, Y., Yoshitake, T., Kato, I., Ohmura, T. *et al.* (1994) 'Changing patterns in the prevalence of dementia in a Japanese community: the Hisayama Study.' *Gerontology 40*, Suppl 2, 29–35.

Knowler, W.C., Fowler, S.E., Hamman, R.F., Christophi, C.A. *et al.* (2009) 'Ten-year follow-up of diabetes incidence and weight loss in the Diabetes Prevention Program Outcomes Study.' *Lancet 374*, 1677–86.

Kramer, A.F., Hahn, S., Cohen, N., Banich, M.T. *et al.* (1999) 'Ageing, fitness and neurocognitive function.' *Nature 400*, 418–19.

Kryscio, R.J., Schmitt, F.A., Salazar, J.C., Mendiondo, M.S. and Markesbery, W.R. (2006) 'Risk factors for transitions from normal to mild cognitive impairment and dementia.' *Neurology 66*, 828–32.

Laitinen, M.H., Ngandu, T., Rovio, S., Helkala, E.L. *et al.* (2006) 'Fat intake at midlife and risk of dementia and Alzheimer's disease: a population-based study.' *Dementia and Geriatric Cognitive Disorders 22*, 99–107.

Larson, E.B., Shadlen, M.F., Wang, L., McCormick, W.C. *et al.* (2004) 'Survival after initial diagnosis of Alzheimer disease.' *Annals of Internal Medicine 140*, 501–9.

Larson, E.B., Wang, L., Bowen, J.D., McCormick, W.C. *et al.* (2006) 'Exercise is associated with reduced risk for incident dementia among persons 65 years of age and older.' *Annals of Internal Medicine 144*, 73–81.

Launer, L.J., Andersen, K., Dewey, M.E., Letenneur, L. *et al.* (1999) 'Rates and risk factors for dementia and Alzheimer's disease: results from EURODEM pooled analyses.' EURODEM Incidence Research Group and Work Groups. European Studies of Dementia. *Neurology 52*, 78–84.

Lautenschlager, N.T., Cox, K.L., Flicker, L., Foster, J.K. *et al.* (2008) 'Effect of physical activity on cognitive function in older adults at risk for Alzheimer disease: a randomized trial.' *Journal of the American Medical Association 300*, 1027–37.

Le Carret, N., Rainville, C., Lechevallier, N., Lafont, S., Letenneur, L. and Fabrigoule, C. (2003) 'Influence of education on the Benton visual retention test performance as mediated by a strategic search component.' *Brain and Cognition 53*, 408–11.

Lee, P.N. (1994) 'Smoking and Alzheimer's disease: a review of the epidemiological evidence.' *Neuroepidemiology 13*, 131–44.

Lemeshow, S., Letenneur, L., Dartigues, J.F., Lafont, S., Orgogozo, J.M. and Commenges, D. (1998) 'Illustration of analysis taking into account complex survey considerations: the association between wine consumption and dementia in the PAQUID study.' *American Journal of Epidemiology 148*, 298–306.

Letenneur, L., Gilleron, V., Commenges, D., Helmer, C., Orgogozo, J.M. and Dartigues, J.F. (1999) 'Are sex and educational level independent predictors of dementia and Alzheimer's disease? Incidence data from the PAQUID project.' *Journal of Neurology, Neurosurgery and Psychiatry 66*, 177–83.

Letenneur, L., Larrieu, S. and Barberger-Gateau, P. (2004) 'Alcohol and tobacco consumption as risk factors of dementia: a review of epidemiological studies.' *Biomedicine and Pharmacotherapy 58*, 95–9.

Letenneur, L., Launer, L.J., Andersen, K., Dewey, M.E. *et al.* (2000) 'Education and the risk for Alzheimer's disease: sex makes a difference.' EURODEM pooled analyses. EURODEM Incidence Research Group. *American Journal of Epidemiology 151*, 1064–71.

Lethaby, A., Hogervorst, E., Richards, M., Yesufu, A. and Yaffe, K. (2008) 'Hormone replacement therapy for cognitive function in postmenopausal women.' *Cochrane Database Syst Rev*, CD003122.

Li, G., Higdon, R., Kukull, W.A., Peskind, E. *et al.* (2004) 'Statin therapy and risk of dementia in the elderly: a community-based prospective cohort study.' *Neurology 63*, 1624–8.

Li, G., Larson, E.B., Sonnen, J.A., Shofer, J.B. *et al.* (2007) 'Statin therapy is associated with reduced neuropathologic changes of Alzheimer disease.' *Neurology 69*, 878–85.

Liu, H.C., Lin, K.N., Teng, E.L., Wang, S.J. *et al.* (1995) 'Prevalence and subtypes of dementia in Taiwan: a community survey of 5297 individuals.' *Journal of the American Geriatrics Society 43*, 144–9.

Lllewellyn, D.J., Lang, I.A., Langa, K.M., Muniz-Terrera, G. *et al.* (2010) 'Vitamin D and risk of cognitive decline in elderly persons.' *Archives of Internal Medicine 170*, 1135–41.

Lobo, A., Launer, L.J., Fratiglioni, L., Andersen, K. *et al.* (2000) 'Prevalence of dementia and major subtypes in Europe: a collaborative study of population-based cohorts.' Neurologic Diseases in the Elderly Research Group. *Neurology 54*, S4–9.

Luchsinger, J.A. (2010) 'Diabetes, related conditions, and dementia.' *Journal of the Neurological Sciences 299*, 1–2, 35–38.

Luchsinger, J.A., Tang, M.X., Miller, J., Green, R. and Mayeux, R. (2007) 'Relation of higher folate intake to lower risk of Alzheimer disease in the elderly.' *Archives of Neurology 64*, 86–92.

Luchsinger, J.A., Tang, M.X., Shea, S., Miller, J., Green, R. and Mayeux, R. (2004) 'Plasma homocysteine levels and risk of Alzheimer disease.' *Neurology 62*, 1972–6.

Lyketsos, C.G., Breitner, J.C., Green, R.C., Martin, B.K. *et al.* (2007) 'Naproxen and celecoxib do not prevent AD in early results from a randomized controlled trial.' *Neurology 68*, 1800–8.

Lytle, M.E., Vander Bilt, J., Pandav, R.S., Dodge, H.H. and Ganguli, M. (2004) 'Exercise level and cognitive decline: the MoVIES project.' *Alzheimer's Disease and Associated Disorders 18*, 57–64.

Maki, P.M. (2006) 'Hormone therapy and cognitive function: is there a critical period for benefit?' *Neuroscience 138*, 1027–30.

Malouf, R. and Grimley Evans, J. (2008) 'Folic acid with or without vitamin B12 for the prevention and treatment of healthy elderly and demented people.' *Cochrane Database Syst Rev*, CD004514.

Manubens, J.M., Martinez-Lage, J.M., Lacruz, F., Muruzabal, J. *et al.* (1995) 'Prevalence of Alzheimer's disease and other dementing disorders in Pamplona, Spain.' *Neuroepidemiology 14*, 155–64.

McGuinness, B., Craig, D., Bullock, R. and Passmore, P. (2009a) 'Statins for the prevention of dementia.' *Cochrane Database Syst Rev*, CD003160.

McGuinness, B., Todd, S., Passmore, P. and Bullock, R. (2009b) 'Blood pressure lowering in patients without prior cerebrovascular disease for prevention of cognitive impairment and dementia.' *Cochrane Database Syst Rev*, CD004034.

McKee, M., Britton, A., Black, N., McPherson, K., Sanderson, C. and Bain, C. (1999) 'Methods in health services research. Interpreting the evidence: choosing between randomised and non-randomised studies.' *British Medical Journal 319*, 312–5.

Merchant, C., Tang, M.X., Albert, S., Manly, J., Stern, Y. and Mayeux, R. (1999) 'The influence of smoking on the risk of Alzheimer's disease.' *Neurology 52*, 1408–12.

Mooijaart, S.P., Gussekloo, J., Frolich, M., Jolles, J. *et al.* (2005) 'Homocysteine, vitamin B-12, and folic acid and the risk of cognitive decline in old age: the Leiden 85-Plus Study.' *American Journal of Clinical Nutrition 82*, 866–71.

Morris, M.C., Evans, D.A., Bienias, J.L., Tangney, C.C. *et al.* (2003a) 'Dietary fats and the risk of incident Alzheimer disease.' *Archives of Neurology 60*, 194–200.

Morris, M.C., Evans, D.A., Bienias, J.L., Tangney, C.C. *et al.* (2003b) 'Consumption of fish and n-3 fatty acids and risk of incident Alzheimer disease.' *Archives of Neurology 60*, 940–6.

Morris, M.C., Evans, D.A., Bienias, J.L., Tangney, C.C. *et al.* (2005a) 'Dietary folate and vitamin B12 intake and cognitive decline among community-dwelling older persons.' *Archives of Neurology 62*, 641–5.

Morris, M.C., Evans, D.A., Schneider, J.A., Tangney, C.C., Bienias, J.L. and Aggarwal, N.T. (2006) 'Dietary folate and vitamins B-12 and B-6 not associated with incident Alzheimer's disease.' *Journal of Alzheimer's Disease 9*, 435–43.

Morris, M.C., Evans, D.A., Tangney, C.C., Bienias, J.L. and Wilson, R.S. (2005b) 'Fish consumption and cognitive decline with age in a large community study.' *Archives of Neurology 62*, 1849–53.

Morris, M.C., Evans, D.A., Tangney, C.C., Bienias, J.L. *et al.* (2005c) 'Relation of the tocopherol forms to incident Alzheimer disease and to cognitive change.' *American Journal of Clinical Nutrition 81*, 508–14.

Mortimer, J.A. and Graves, A.B. (1993) 'Education and other socioeconomic determinants of dementia and Alzheimer's disease.' *Neurology 43*, S39–S44.

O'Connor, D.W., Pollitt, P.A. and Treasure, F.P. (1991) 'The influence of education and social class on the diagnosis of dementia in a community population.' *Psychological Medicine 21*, 219–24.

Oken, B.S., Zajdel, D., Kishiyama, S., Flegal, K. *et al.* (2006) 'Randomized, controlled, six-month trial of yoga in healthy seniors: effects on cognition and quality of life.' *Alternative Therapies in Health and Medicine 12*, 40–7.

Ott, A., Andersen, K., Dewey, M.E., Letenneur, L. *et al.* (2004) 'Effect of smoking on global cognitive function in nondemented elderly.' *Neurology 62*, 920–4.

Ott, A., Breteler, M.M., Van Harskamp, F., Claus, J.J. *et al.* (1995) 'Prevalence of Alzheimer's disease and vascular dementia: association with education. The Rotterdam Study.' *British Medical Journal 310*, 970–3.

Ott, A., Slooter, A.J., Hofman, A., Van Harskamp, F. *et al.* (1998) 'Smoking and risk of dementia and Alzheimer's disease in a population-based cohort study: the Rotterdam Study.' *Lancet 351*, 1840–3.

Peters, R., Peters, J., Warner, J., Beckett, N. and Bulpitt, C. (2008) 'Alcohol, dementia and cognitive decline in the elderly: a systematic review.' *Age and Ageing 37*, 505–12.

Pfeffer, R.I., Afifi, A.A. and Chance, J.M. (1987) 'Prevalence of Alzheimer's disease in a retirement community.' *American Journal of Epidemiology 125*, 420–36.

Podewils, L.J., Guallar, E., Kuller, L.H., Fried, L.P. *et al.* (2005) 'Physical activity, APOE genotype, and dementia risk: findings from the Cardiovascular Health Cognition Study.' *American Journal of Epidemiology 161*, 639–51.

Polo-Kantola, P., Portin, R., Polo, O., Helenius, H., Irjala, K. and Erkkola, R. (1998) 'The effect of short-term estrogen replacement therapy on cognition: a randomized, double-blind, cross-over trial in postmenopausal women.' *Obstetrics and Gynecology 91*, 459–66.

Potter, G.G., Helms, M.J. and Plassman, B.L. (2008) 'Associations of job demands and intelligence with cognitive performance among men in late life.' *Neurology 70*, 1803–8.

Prencipe, M., Casini, A.R., Ferretti, C., Lattanzio, M.T., Fiorelli, M. and Culasso, F. (1996) 'Prevalence of dementia in an elderly rural population: effects of age, sex, and education.' *Journal of Neurology, Neurosurgery and Psychiatry 60*, 628–33.

Prince, M., Cullen, M. and Mann, A. (1994) 'Risk factors for Alzheimer's disease and dementia: A case-control study based on the MRC elderly hypertension trial.' *Neurology 44*, 97–104.

Qiu, C., Winblad, B. and Fratiglioni, L. (2005) 'The age-dependent relation of blood pressure to cognitive function and dementia.' *Lancet Neurology 4*, 487–99.

Qiu, C., Winblad, B. and Fratiglioni, L. (2009) 'Low diastolic pressure and risk of dementia in very old people: a longitudinal study.' *Dementia and Geriatric Cognitive Disorders 28*, 213–19.

Ravaglia, G., Forti, P., Maioli, F., Martelli, M. *et al.* (2005) 'Homocysteine and folate as risk factors for dementia and Alzheimer disease.' *American Journal of Clinical Nutrition 82*, 636–43.

Ravaglia, G., Forti, P., Maioli, F., Sacchetti, L. *et al.* (2002) 'Education, occupation, and prevalence of dementia: findings from the Conselice study.' *Dementia and Geriatric Cognitive Disorders 14*, 90–100.

Rea, T.D., Breitner, J.C., Psaty, B.M., Fitzpatrick, A.L. *et al.* (2005) 'Statin use and the risk of incident dementia: the Cardiovascular Health Study.' *Archives of Neurology 62*, 1047–51.

Richard, E., Van Den Heuvel, E., Moll Van Charante, E.P., Achthoven, L. *et al.* (2009) 'Prevention of dementia by intensive vascular care (PreDIVA): a cluster-randomized trial in progress.' *Alzheimer's Disease and Associated Disorders 23*, 198–204.

Richards, M., Shipley, B., Fuhrer, R. and Wadsworth, M.E. (2004) 'Cognitive ability in childhood and cognitive decline in mid-life: longitudinal birth cohort study.' *British Medical Journal 328*, 552.

Riggs, J.E. (1993) 'Smoking and Alzheimer's disease: protective effect or differential survival bias? *Lancet 342*, 793–4.

Rocca, W.A., Van Duijn, C.M., Clayton, D., Chandra, V. *et al.* (1991) 'Maternal age and Alzheimer's disease: a collaborative re-analysis of case-control studies.' EURODEM Risk Factors Research Group. *International Journal of Epidemiology 20*, Suppl 2, S21–7.

Rockwood, K., Kirkland, S., Hogan, D.B., Macknight, C. *et al.* (2002) 'Use of lipid-lowering agents, indication bias, and the risk of dementia in community-dwelling elderly people.' *Archives of Neurology 59*, 223–7.

Saczynski, J.S., Pfeifer, L.A., Masaki, K., Korf, E.S. *et al.* (2006) 'The effect of social engagement on incident dementia: the Honolulu–Asia Aging Study.' *American Journal of Epidemiology 163*, 433–40.

Satz, P., Morgenstern, H., Miller, E.N., Selnes, O.A. *et al.* (1993) 'Low education as a possible risk factor for cognitive abnormalities in HIV-1: findings from the Multicenter AIDS Cohort Study (MACS).' *Journal of Acquired Immune Deficiency Syndrome 6*, 503–11.

Savaskan, E., Olivieri, G., Meier, F., Seifritz, E., Wirz-Justice, A. and Muller-Spahn, F. (2003) 'Red wine ingredient resveratrol protects from beta-amyloid neurotoxicity.' *Gerontology 49*, 380–3.

Scarmeas, N., Levy, G., Tang, M.X., Manly, J. and Stern, Y. (2001) 'Influence of leisure activity on the incidence of Alzheimer's disease.' *Neurology 57*, 2236–42.

Scarmeas, N., Luchsinger, J.A., Schupf, N., Brickman, A.M. *et al.* (2009) 'Physical activity, diet, and risk of Alzheimer disease.' *Journal of the American Medical Association 302*, 627–37.

Scarmeas, N., Stern, Y., Tang, M.X., Mayeux, R. and Luchsinger, J.A. (2006) 'Mediterranean diet and risk for Alzheimer's disease.' *Annals of Neurology 59*, 912–21.

Schaefer, E.J., Bongard, V., Beiser, A.S., Lamon-Fava, S. *et al.* (2006) 'Plasma phosphatidylcholine docosahexaenoic acid content and risk of dementia and Alzheimer disease: the Framingham Heart Study.' *Archives of Neurology 63*, 1545–50.

Seshadri, S., Beiser, A., Selhub, J., Jacques, P.F. *et al.* (2002) 'Plasma homocysteine as a risk factor for dementia and Alzheimer's disease.' *New England Journal of Medicine 346*, 476–83.

Shumaker, S.A., Legault, C., Kuller, L., Rapp, S.R. *et al.* (2004) 'Conjugated equine estrogens and incidence of probable dementia and mild cognitive impairment in postmenopausal women: Women's Health Initiative Memory Study.' *Journal of the American Medical Association 291*, 2947–58.

Shumaker, S.A., Legault, C., Rapp, S.R., Thal, L. *et al.* (2003) 'Estrogen plus progestin and the incidence of dementia and mild cognitive impairment in postmenopausal women. The Women's Health Initiative Memory Study: a randomized controlled trial.' *Journal of the American Medical Association 289*, 2651–62.

Skoog, I., Nilsson, L., Palmeritz, B., Andreasson, L.A. and Svanborg, A. (1993) 'A population-based study of dementia in 85-year-olds.' *New England Journal of Medicine 328*, 153–8.

Slinin, Y., Paudel, M.L., Taylor, B.C., Fink, H.A. *et al.* (2010) '25-Hydroxyvitamin D levels and cognitive performance and decline in elderly men.' *Neurology 74*, 33–41.

Sofi, F., Valecchi, D., Bacci, D., Abbate, R. *et al.* (2011) 'Physical activity and risk of cognitive decline: a meta-analysis of prospective studies.' *Journal of Internal Medicine 269*, 107–17.

Solfrizzi, V., Colacicco, A.M., D'Introno, A., Capurso, C. *et al.* (2006a) 'Dietary fatty acids intakes and rate of mild cognitive impairment: the Italian Longitudinal Study on Aging.' *Experimental Gerontology 41*, 619–27.

Solfrizzi, V., Colacicco, A.M., D'Introno, A., Capurso, C. *et al.* (2006b) 'Dietary intake of unsaturated fatty acids and age-related cognitive decline: a 8.5-year follow-up of the Italian Longitudinal Study on Aging.' *Neurobiology of Aging 27*, 1694–704.

Stern, Y. (2006) 'Cognitive reserve and Alzheimer disease.' *Alzheimer's Disease and Associated Disorders 20*, 112–17.

Stern, Y., Alexander, G.E., Prohovnik, I. and Mayeux, R. (1992) 'Inverse relationship between education and parietotemporal perfusion deficit in Alzheimer's disease.' *Annals of Neurology 32*, 371–5.

Stern, Y., Gurland, B., Tatemichi, T.K., Tang, M.X., Wilder, D. and Mayeux, R. (1994) 'Influence of education and occupation on the incidence of Alzheimer's disease.' *Journal of the American Medical Association 271*, 1004–10.

Sulkava, R., Wikstrom, J., Aromaa, A., Raitasalo, R. *et al.* (1985) 'Prevalence of severe dementia in Finland.' *Neurology 35*, 1025–9.

Szekely, C.A., Thorne, J.E., Zandi, P.P., Ek, M. *et al.* (2004) 'Nonsteroidal anti-inflammatory drugs for the prevention of Alzheimer's disease: a systematic review.' *Neuroepidemiology 23*, 159–69.

Teunissen, C.E., Blom, A.H., Van Boxtel, M.P., Bosma, H. *et al.* (2003) 'Homocysteine: A marker for cognitive performance? A longitudinal follow-up study.' *Journal of Nutrition, Health and Aging 7*, 153–9.

Tucker, K.L., Qiao, N., Scott, T., Rosenberg, I. and Spiro, A. 3rd (2005) 'High homocysteine and low B vitamins predict cognitive decline in aging men: the Veterans Affairs Normative Aging Study.' *American Journal of Clinical Nutrition 82*, 627–35.

Tuomilehto, J., Lindstrom, J., Eriksson, J.G., Valle, T.T. *et al.* (2001) 'Prevention of type 2 diabetes mellitus by changes in lifestyle among subjects with impaired glucose tolerance.' *New England Journal of Medicine 344*, 1343–50.

t' Veld, B.A., Ruitenberg, A., Hofman, A., Launer, L.J. *et al.* (2001) 'Nonsteroidal antiinflammatory drugs and the risk of Alzheimer's disease.' *New England Journal of Medicine 345*, 1515–21.

Van Duijn, C.M., Clayton, D.G., Chandra, V., Fratiglioni, L. *et al.* (1994) 'Interaction between genetic and environmental risk factors for Alzheimer's disease: a re-analysis of case-control studies.' EURODEM Risk Factors Research Group. *Genetic Epidemiology 11*, 539–51.

Van Gelder, B.M., Tijhuis, M., Kalmijn, S. and Kromhout, D. (2007) 'Fish consumption, n-3 fatty acids, and subsequent 5-y cognitive decline in elderly men: the Zutphen Elderly Study.' *American Journal of Clinical Nutrition 85*, 1142–7.

Van Gelder, B.M., Tijhuis, M.A., Kalmijn, S., Giampaoli, S., Nissinen, A. and Kromhout, D. (2004) 'Physical activity in relation to cognitive decline in elderly men: the FINE Study.' *Neurology 63*, 2316–21.

Verghese, J., Levalley, A., Derby, C., Kuslansky, G. *et al.* (2006) 'Leisure activities and the risk of amnestic mild cognitive impairment in the elderly.' *Neurology 66*, 821–7.

Verghese, J., Lipton, R.B., Katz, M.J., Hall, C.B. *et al.* (2003) 'Leisure activities and the risk of dementia in the elderly.' *New England Journal of Medicine 348*, 2508–16.

Viscoli, C.M., Brass, L.M., Kernan, W.N., Sarrel, P.M., Suissa, S. and Horwitz, R.I. (2005) 'Estrogen therapy and risk of cognitive decline: results from the Women's Estrogen for Stroke Trial (WEST).' *American Journal of Obstetrics and Gynecology 192*, 387–93.

Wang, H.X., Karp, A., Winblad, B. and Fratiglioni, L. (2002) 'Late-life engagement in social and leisure activities is associated with a decreased risk of dementia: a longitudinal study from the Kungsholmen project.' *American Journal of Epidemiology 155*, 1081–7.

Wang, H.X., Wahlin, A., Basun, H., Fastbom, J., Winblad, B. and Fratiglioni, L. (2001) 'Vitamin B(12) and folate in relation to the development of Alzheimer's disease.' *Neurology 56*, 1188–94.

Wang, J.Y., Zhou, D.H., Li, J., Zhang, M. *et al.* (2006) 'Leisure activity and risk of cognitive impairment: the Chongqing aging study.' *Neurology 66*, 911–13.

Wesnes, K.A., Ward, T., McGinty, A. and Petrini, O. (2000) 'The memory enhancing effects of a Ginkgo biloba/Panax ginseng combination in healthy middle-aged volunteers.' *Psychopharmacology (Berl) 152*, 353–61.

Weuve, J., Kang, J.H., Manson, J.E., Bretler, M.M., Ware, J.H. and Grodstein, F. (2004) 'Physical activity, including walking, and cognitive function in older women.' *Journal of the American Medical Association 292*, 1454–61.

Whalley, L.J., Dick, F.D. and McNeill, G. (2006) 'A life-course approach to the aetiology of late-onset dementias.' *Lancet Neurology 5*, 87–96.

Williamson, J.D., Miller, M.E., Bryan, R.N., Lazar, R.M. *et al.* (2007) 'The Action to Control Cardiovascular Risk in Diabetes Memory in Diabetes Study (ACCORD-MIND): rationale, design, and methods.' *American Journal of Cardiology 99*, 112i–122i.

Willis, S.L., Tennstedt, S.L., Marsiske, M., Ball, K. *et al.* (2006) 'Long-term effects of cognitive training on everyday functional outcomes in older adults.' *Journal of the American Medical Association 296*, 2805–14.

Wilson, R.S., Bennett, D.A., Bienias, J.L., Aggarwal, N.T. *et al.* (2002a) 'Cognitive activity and incident AD in a population-based sample of older persons.' *Neurology 59*, 1910–14.

Wilson, R.S., Bennett, D.A., Bienias, J.L., Mendes De Leon, C.F. *et al.* (2003) 'Cognitive activity and cognitive decline in a biracial community population.' *Neurology 61*, 812–16.

Wilson, R.S., Krueger, K.R., Kamenetsky, J.M., Tang, Y. *et al.* (2005a) 'Hallucinations and mortality in Alzheimer disease.' *American Journal of Geriatric Psychiatry 13*, 984–90.

Wilson, R.S., Mendes De Leon, C.F., Barnes, L.L., Schneider, J.A. *et al.* (2002b) 'Participation in cognitively stimulating activities and risk of incident Alzheimer disease.' *Journal of the American Medical Association 287*, 742–8.

Wilson, R.S., Scherr, P.A., Bienias, J.L., Mendes De Leon, C.F. (2005b) 'Socioeconomic characteristics of the community in childhood and cognition in old age.' *Experimental Aging Research 31*, 393–407.

Wilson, R.S., Scherr, P.A., Schneider, J.A., Tang, Y. and Bennett, D.A. (2007) 'Relation of cognitive activity to risk of developing Alzheimer disease.' *Neurology 69*, 1911–20.

Wolozin, B., Kellman, W., Ruosseau, P., Celesia, G.G. and Siegel, G. (2000) 'Decreased prevalence of Alzheimer disease associated with 3-hydroxy-3-methyglutaryl coenzyme A reductase inhibitors.' *Archives of Neurology 57*, 1439–43.

Woo, J.I., Lee, J.H., Yoo, K.Y., Kim, C.Y., Kim, Y.I. and Shin, Y.S. (1998) 'Prevalence estimation of dementia in a rural area of Korea.' *Journal of the American Geriatrics Society 46*, 983–7.

Yaffe, K., Barnes, D., Nevitt, M., Lui, L.Y. and Covinsky, K. (2001) 'A prospective study of physical activity and cognitive decline in elderly women: women who walk.' *Archives of Internal Medicine 161*, 1703–8.

Yaffe, K., Barrett-Connor, E., Lin, F. and Grady, D. (2002) 'Serum lipoprotein levels, statin use, and cognitive function in older women.' *Archives of Neurology 59*, 378–84.

Yaffe, K., Clemons, T.E., McBee, W.L. and Linblad, A.S. (2004) 'Impact of antioxidants, zinc, and copper on cognition in the elderly: a randomized, controlled trial.' *Neurology 63*, 1705–7.

Yamada, M., Sasaki, H., Mimori, Y., Kasagi, F. *et al.* (1999) 'Prevalence and risks of dementia in the Japanese population: RERF's adult health study Hiroshima subjects. Radiation Effects Research Foundation.' *Journal of the American Geriatrics Society 47*, 189–95.

Yoshitake, T., Kiyohara, Y., Kato, I., Ohmura, T. *et al.* (1995) 'Incidence and risk factors of vascular dementia and Alzheimer's disease in a defined elderly Japanese population: the Hisayama Study.' *Neurology 45*, 1161–8.

Zandi, P.P., Sparks, D.L., Khachaturian, A.S., Tschanz, J. *et al.* (2005) 'Do statins reduce risk of incident dementia and Alzheimer disease? The Cache County Study.' *Archives of General Psychiatry 62*, 217–24.

Zhou, D.F., Wu, C.S., Qi, H., Fan, J.H. *et al.* (2006) 'Prevalence of dementia in rural China: impact of age, gender and education.' *Acta Neurologica Scandinavica 114*, 273–80.

Chapter 4

Integrated Care and Treatment of Dementia

Defining Best Practice for the Twenty-first Century

Laura Telford, Emily Gallagher and Emma Reynish

Context

The framework of strategy and policy that currently exists for guiding the care and treatment of people with dementia is diverse. At an international level numerous countries have 'dementia plans' or strategies (Alzheimer Europe 2010). In the UK, national dementia strategies exist for the four devolved nations. All are slightly different but each recognises the importance of maintaining independence and dignity for people with dementia, the importance of valuing informal caregivers, the importance of an early diagnosis, and the importance of improving the general hospital response to dementia. In addition to these national dementia plans, individual patient organisations (international and national) assume the role that defines and advocates 'good practice' for this population and their carers. Policy and practice in this area are also guided by organisations with a remit to cover more specific areas of practice. For example, in the UK the National Institute of Clinical Excellence (NICE) assimilates clinical evidence to publish guidelines on specific areas of treatment and practice. Professional organisations produce guidance and campaign on specific areas of practice – for example, the British Geriatrics Society 'Do not forget the person' campaign (British Geriatrics Society 2010). The National Care Forum has produced 'Key principles of person-centred dementia care' (National Care Forum 2007), and in Scotland the Mental Welfare Commission works to safeguard the rights and welfare of those with dementia. In addition, results of specific research projects in a diverse range of areas concerning dementia, from brain cell pathology (Hyman *et al.* 1984) to music therapy (Nair *et al.* 2011), are published in a multitude of academic journals each year and form the essential platform from which future evidence-based policy is drawn.

Despite this wealth of guidance, the treatment, management and care for people with dementia is often seen as polarised, with the two polarities seen as mutually exclusive. On the one hand the biomedical approach has traditionally been the default health care delivery. Research in this field is typified by large randomised controlled trials of single treatments for one pathological process, for example Alzheimer's disease. The opposite end of the spectrum is typified by the psychosocial approach – traditionally the domain of social care. Research in this field is social-science based and person-centred, covering a more true-to-life homogeneous population. By starting with an understanding of patient and caregiver expectations, it is possible to blur the boundaries between these traditional approaches to dementia treatment and care. The aim of this chapter is therefore to describe truly 'person-centred biomedical treatment' (the dawn of the concept of multicomponent intervention for dementia) that defines best practice for dementia treatment and care at the beginning of the twenty-first century.

Understanding expectations

People with dementia and their carers have different experiences of dementia, depending on many factors, including physical and emotional well-being, and the support available to them. With the recent publication of national dementia strategies in the UK, more has been documented formally about the expectations and rights of individuals with dementia and their carers. In England the document *Quality Outcomes for People with Dementia* (Department of Health 2010) states that by 2014, all people living with dementia in England should be able to say:

- I was diagnosed early.
- I understand, so I make good decisions and provide for future decision making.
- I get the treatment and support which are best for my dementia, and my life.
- Those around me and looking after me are well supported.
- I am treated with dignity and respect.
- I know what I can do to help myself and who else can help me.
- I can enjoy life.
- I feel part of a community and I'm inspired to give something back.
- I am confident my end of life wishes will be respected. I can expect a good death.

In Scotland the charter of rights for people with dementia (Dementia Rights 2009) states that:

> People with dementia and their carers have…the right to live as independently as possible…the right to full participation in care needs assessment, planning, deciding and arranging care, support and treatment, including advanced decision making…
>
> Public and private bodies, voluntary organisations and individuals responsible for the care and treatment of persons with dementia should be held accountable for the respect, protection and fulfilment of their human rights…
>
> People with dementia have the right to help to attain and maintain maximum independence, physical, mental, social and vocational ability, and full inclusion and participation in all aspects of life…

The opinions expressed in both documents build a very clear picture of desired outcomes for the treatment and care that come from across the spectrum of biomedical and psychosocial models of care.

Changes in the delivery of treatment for the population with dementia have been hampered by lack of robust clinical evidence for definite, effective, pharmacological treatment. This does not, however, imply that intervention does not work, but rather does reflect the complex nature of dementia, resulting in difficulty developing methodologies when planning rigorous scientific research. Given the heterogeneous nature of the population with dementia (a syndrome rather than single disease entity) and the wide-ranging positive outcomes that could be expected, it is complexity that hampers the documentation of such evidence. Despite this complexity, increasing evidence does exist which is starting to link what appears to be best practice with desired outcomes for patients and carers, that is, intervention is being shown to deliver on patient expectations. For example, carer support and counselling at diagnosis can reduce care home placement by 28 per cent (Mittelman 2007). Early diagnosis and intervention has been shown to improve the quality of life of people with dementia (Banerjee *et al.* 2007), and early intervention has positive effects on the quality of life of family carers (Mittelman 2007).

Understanding the population with dementia

Who has dementia?

In addition to understanding the desired meaningful outcomes that could make a difference to the lives of those affected with dementia, it is important to understand patient needs at a population level. The European Collaboration on Dementia (EuroCoDe) was developed in order to recognise the global impact of dementia (Alzheimer Europe 2010).

By looking at the prevalence of a disease in a population it is possible to define the parts of the population that are affected by that disease and make estimates of the service needed to deliver treatment and care to the affected population.

The prevalence part of the EuroCoDe project involved a systematic review of all epidemiological studies carried out in Europe after 1991, followed by a collaborative analysis of raw data obtained from these studies, thereby enabling a comparison of results with the EURODEM study (Hofman *et al.* 1991), which had collected data from studies carried out before the 1990s. Results are shown in Table 4.1 and graphically in Figure 4.1.

Table 4.1 Prevalence of dementia comparing sexes within different age groups

Age	Male % prevalence	Female % prevalence
60–64	0.2	0.9
65–69	1.8	1.4
70–74	3.2	3.8
75–79	7.0	7.6
80–84	14.5	16.4
85–89	20.9	28.5
90–94	29.2	44.4
>95	32.4	48.8

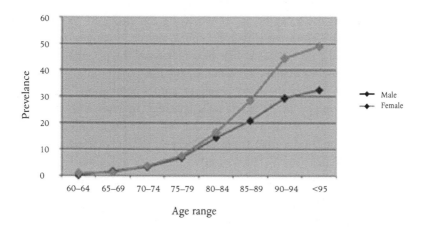

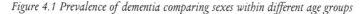

Figure 4.1 Prevalence of dementia comparing sexes within different age groups

Comparison with the prevalence rate from the EURODEM and EuroCoDe studies shows that dementia prevalence has not changed since the 1990s. However, with the advent of recent studies measuring prevalence in the 'oldest old', prevalence rates may have been under-reported in this age group. As can be seen in Figure 4.1, in the female population aged over 95, individuals have a one in two chance of having dementia.

What does this prevalence mean in terms of numbers of people affected? By mapping these prevalence figures onto known population data it is possible to get an estimate of the numbers of people with dementia. To illustrate this we have used the Scottish population (General Register Office for Scotland 2010) in Figure 4.2.

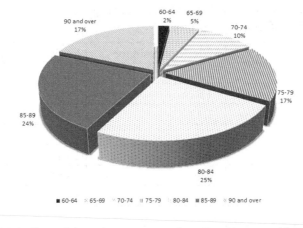

Figure 4.2 Incidence of dementia per age group from 60 to 90+ years old

From this we can see that approximately two-thirds of the population with dementia are over the age of 80 and a significant number are over 90. This in not surprising when aging is known to be the strongest risk factor for dementia (Evans 1996), but it does set the scene for looking at the delivery of treatment and care for dementia: the majority of the population needing treatment and care for dementia will come from the 'oldest old' part of society. It also follows that, with an increasingly aging population, the absolute numbers of people with dementia will continue to rise, with predictions that the worldwide prevalence of dementia will increase by 85 per cent by the year 2030 and more than triple by the year 2050 (Alzheimer's Disease International 2010).

Young onset dementia

Epidemiological data for prevalence rates for young onset dementia is sparse, and methods of case ascertainment vary between studies. At a population level, young onset dementia remains a rare condition with relatively low case numbers. At an individual level the impact of the disease can be catastrophic. Patients with early onset dementia have similar care needs to older patients, but a younger person with dementia may, for example, have dependent children, be in work at the time of diagnosis, have heavy financial commitments, find it difficult to rationalise losing skills at such a young age, and find it difficult to access appropriate information and support (Alzheimer's Society 2002). Because of this the impact that the disabilities associated with early onset dementia have on an individual's autonomy and quality of life is significant.

How many people are diagnosed with dementia?

As we have seen, in older age dementia is relatively common and there is a well-documented discrepancy between those people who exhibit one or many of the symptoms of dementia but do not have a formal diagnosis, and those who, in response to their symptoms, receive a formal diagnosis. This difference has been termed the 'dementia gap' in a recent report published by Tesco and the national Alzheimer Societies in England and Scotland (Alzheimer's Society 2011a). This has been documented numerically for the British population by comparing the numbers predicted to have dementia, based on prevalence data and each local population, and the number of those who do have a formal diagnosis of dementia, which is obtained from GP registers (Quality Outcome Framework [QOF] targets). From this exercise the predicted diagnostic gap for all regions has been published and shows a gradient from 69 per cent with a diagnosis, down to 27 per cent with a diagnosis in some regions. Looking in more detail at this diagnostic gap, a recent cohort study of dementia prevalence in the acute hospital setting (Sampson et al. 2009) showed that of the older population 42 per cent had dementia, but of these half did not have a formal diagnosis. From the same study, Table 4.2 shows the prevalence of dementia in the acute hospital setting. It shows a higher prevalence in the hospital setting than in the general population, which confirms that those with minor illness and dementia are more likely to require emergency treatment in hospital. It can be seen in addition that prevalence rises with age in parallel with prevalence shown for the general population, with, once again, the 'oldest old' suffering most frequently with dementia.

Table 4.2 Prevalence of dementia within the acute hospital setting

Age	Male % prevalence	Female % prevalence
70–79 years	16.4	29.6
>90 years	48.8	75.0

HOW IMPORTANT IS IT AT AN INDIVIDUAL LEVEL TO HAVE A FORMAL DIAGNOSIS OF DEMENTIA?

The voices of all national and international disease societies are in agreement about the advantage achieved by a formal diagnosis (Alzheimer's Association 2009), and there is now increasing evidence that a variety of interventions at an early stage can improve outcomes (DeKosky 2003; Moniz-Cook *et al.* 1998), despite continuing lack of definite disease-modifying pharmaceutical intervention for any of the dementia subtypes. Public opinion mirrors this, with results of an international survey showing that over 85 per cent of respondents in the five countries surveyed said that if they were exhibiting confusion and memory loss, they would want to see a doctor to determine whether the cause of the symptoms was Alzheimer's disease or related disease. In addition, over 94 per cent would want the same if a family member were exhibiting the symptoms (Blendon *et al.* 2011).

With the consensus being that a formal diagnosis is advantageous, we must ask what the barriers are that hamper our ability to improve diagnostic rates. There is a feeling amongst health care professionals that lack of presentation to the health care system is the main barrier. Reasons for this are numerous: symptoms may be perceived as 'normal aging'; symptoms may be thought of as atypical (e.g. failing to be able to perform everyday activities at home); 'physical symptoms' may predominate (e.g. poor mobility and falls); and there may be sudden deterioration associated with mild illness, or even no definite memory problem. On occasions the explanation may be simpler, due to lack of a caregiver to raise awareness. Fear of the diagnosis plays a significant part in this scenario, and will continue to be a major setback until the public portrayal of dementia is modified from a condition for which 'nothing can be done' to one in which early diagnosis results in advantageous outcomes for individuals and their caregivers.

The recent changes in the UK to NICE technology appraisal numbers 217 and 210 (NICE 2011a, 2011b; see Box 4.1 and Box 4.2 on pages 93 and 94) may help to change public opinion, with advice now soundly suggesting a viable treatment option for all stages of Alzheimer's disease, and a treatment to prevent secondary stroke disease that is a viable option for those with vascular dementia. The public message, therefore, from this national guidance is that treatment options do now exist for all stages of Alzheimer's disease and vascular dementia, and dementia is no longer a condition for which 'nothing can be done'.

What are the treatment and care needs of the population with dementia?

Symptoms of dementia and their treatment

Dementia is classically perceived as a condition characterised by memory loss. In addition to this cognitive decline, many other problems may be associated with this disease, including functional decline, neuropsychiatric symptoms and caregiver burden.

Memory loss (amnesic cognitive decline) is generally a salient feature but is often accompanied, or even predated, by a number of co-existing symptoms. There is often loss of ability in other cognitive domains such as executive functioning (an ability to process complex tasks) and language.

In other instances gradual functional decline (ability to perform everyday activities) may be apparent, evidenced by, for example, failing ability to continue to manage domestic finances, reduced aptitude with familiar recipes in the kitchen, or inability to continue using normal modes of transport, etc. In some instances these signs may be attributed to advancing age rather than a disease process, therefore delaying the diagnosis of dementia.

Neuropsychiatric symptoms vary in prevalence throughout the course of disease (Craig *et al.* 2005) and cover a range of symptoms, from apathy to the more frightening behavioural disturbance which – rarely – results in psychotic symptoms associated with dementia.

CAREGIVER BURDEN

In addition to the symptoms experienced by the individual with dementia, the effect on caregivers must also be considered. Taking care of a patient with dementia is known to be stressful, and caregivers often experience high levels of burden (George *et al.* 1986). The caregiver's burden is defined as 'the physical, psychological or emotional, social and financial problems that can be experienced by family members caring for impaired elderly adults' (Pinquart 2003). The burden has both objective and subjective components. Those caring for people with dementia are likely to experience psychological distress (Cohen *et al.* 1990) and depressive symptoms (Covinsky *et al.* 2003); to feel isolated (Schulz *et al.* 1995; Williamson *et al.* 1993); and to have an increased risk of physical health problems (Kiecolt-Glaser *et al.* 1991; King *et al.* 1994) and of dying (Schulz *et al.* 1999). Furthermore, studies have concluded that caregivers are more likely to experience work disruption, health problems and strain than other carers (Ory *et al.* 1999). This array of symptoms must not be overlooked when planning treatment and care in dementia.

Temporal nature of the symptoms of dementia

At any one stage of the disease, an individual may have one or many of the typical symptoms of dementia. Figure 4.3 represents the typical change in these symptoms with time and highlights their fluctuating nature through the course of the disease.

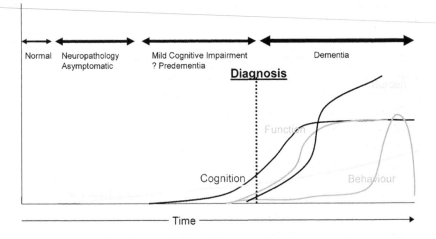

Figure 4.3 Dementia: spectrum of symptoms over the course of the disease

Treatment and care

The importance of the individual and putting them at the centre of their treatment and care should be embedded throughout all stages of dementia. This means helping the person feel valued, acting with courtesy, respecting privacy, and supporting their carers. Often the ways problems present will depend very much on patients' personality, on their relationships with others, and on who they are. People with dementia have had a full and varied life prior to its development, and it is important always to remember this when providing care. This approach has often been termed 'person-centred care' following the work of Tom Kitwood and colleagues (Kitwood 1993). People with dementia should have the opportunity to make informed decisions about their care and treatment. If they do not have the capacity to make decisions, the Mental Capacity Act (England) or equivalent should be used to provide the conditions in which person-centred care can be delivered.

TREATMENT OF ALZHEIMER'S DISEASE

The evidence for the treatment of the symptoms of Alzheimer's disease is well established. Acetyl cholinesterase inhibitors (ACHE I) have been shown to have had a significant beneficial effect on cognitive function and functional ability for some time (Birks 2006; Mulsant *et al.* 2003). In the UK, recent changes in NICE guidance have suggested that they do afford a cost benefit for mild to moderate disease and they are therefore recommended for routine treatment of Alzheimer's disease from its earliest stages. The N-methyl D-aspartate (NMDA) receptor antagonist memantine has been shown to have positive effects in relation to cognitive function, functional ability, delayed need for full-time care, and to a lesser degree neuropsychiatric disturbance in Alzheimer's disease (Reisberg *et al.* 2003). Following recent changes to NICE guidance, memantine is now recommended for the treatment of moderate Alzheimer's disease in cases where ACHE I are contraindicated, and for severe Alzheimer's disease. Box 4.1 shows the summary of the NICE guidance.

Box 4.1 Summary of NICE technology appraisal guidance 217

- Specifically:
  - donepezil, galantamine and rivastigmine are now recommended as options for managing *mild* as well as *moderate* AD
  - memantine is now recommended as an option for managing moderate Alzheimer's disease for people who cannot take ACHE I and as an option for managing *severe* AD.
- Treatment should be continued when it is considered to be having a worthwhile effect on cognitive, global, functional or behavioural symptoms.

The impact of this guidance on practice is significant and means that at every stage of AD there is evidence for symptomatic treatment, which is now supported by clinical guidance from NICE.

TREATMENT OF VASCULAR DEMENTIA

The treatment of vascular dementia is less well defined, in part due to unclear neuropathological classification of underlying aetiology. Vascular disease of the brain associated with cognitive impairment can be seen to cover an extensive spectrum. This starts with overt stroke disease (large vessel occlusive disease) which results in post-stroke dementia, through to covert (absent typical stroke symptoms) stroke disease with lacunar cerebral infarcts caused by occlusive smaller vessel disease, and finishes with 'diffuse periventricular small vessel disease', the patho-physiology of which remains unclear.

The association of dementia *per se* with vascular risk is well documented (Kivipelto *et al.* 2001) in epidemiological studies, but the idea of modifying vascular risk as a treatment for dementia is lacking definite evidence.

It is, however, generally accepted that, in individuals with significant vascular risk (high blood pressure, diabetes, smoking), whether they have dementia or not, active management of these vascular risks is of clinical importance for general health and well-being.

Data on the secondary prevention of stroke disease is, however, robust (Heart Protection Study Collaborative Group 2002; PROGRESS Collaborative Group 2001). The evidence for secondary prevention of stroke disease is well documented and has recently culminated in a change in NICE guidance for the treatment of occlusive vascular disease (NICE 2011a).

Treatments for secondary prevention of stroke disease were poorly tolerated in the elderly population, with dipyridamole causing lowering of the blood pressure and increasing likelihood of dizziness and falls, resulting in withholding or withdrawal of treatment. Clopidogrel alone (rather than aspirin and dipyridamole) is now recommended. The lack of significant side-effects of clopidogrel compared to dipyridamole is of huge clinical significance for the population with vascular dementia, and has resulted in a viable treatment option in vascular dementia. Box 4.2 shows the summary of the NICE guidance.

Box 4.2 Summary of NICE technology appraisal guidance 210

1. *Clopidogrel* is recommended as an option to prevent occlusive vascular events:
   - for people who have had an ischaemic stroke or who have peripheral arterial disease or multi-vascular disease
   - for people who have had a myocardial infarction only if aspirin is contraindicated or not tolerated.

2. Modified-release *dipyridamole in combination with aspirin* is recommended as an option to prevent occlusive vascular events:
   - for people who have had a transient ischaemic attack
   - for people who have had an ischaemic stroke only if clopidogrel is contraindicated or not tolerated.

In stroke disease associated with atrial fibrillation (AF), treatment with anti-coagulation has been shown to prevent the occurrence of further strokes (Stroke

Prevention in Atrial Fibrillation investigators 1991, 1994, 1996). In patients with vascular dementia due to stroke disease and AF, the risks and benefits of their treatment with anti-coagulation should be carefully considered, with recurrent falls often being seen as a contraindication to treatment. With careful treatment monitoring, the potential to prevent loss of independence in those with mild to moderate dementia is, however, considerate.

Unfortunately, secondary prevention in vascular dementia due to covert stroke disease (often seen as lacunar infarcts on brain imaging without typical features of stroke other than cognitive deficits) remains poorly researched. In hospital clinical practice, experts in vascular cognitive impairment and many stroke physicians suggest that this clinical picture should be viewed as occlusive vascular disease and therefore treated with secondary prevention with clopidogrel.

The management of 'diffuse vascular small vessel disease' requires further study. Patients should receive appropriate management of vascular risk factors for their general health and well-being.

TREATMENT OF NEUROPSYCHIATRIC SYMPTOMS

The management and treatment of neuropsychiatric symptoms associated with dementia has been frequently discussed due to the prevalent use of anti-psychotic medication for symptom control, which has been shown to be associated with poor patient outcomes and increased mortality (Schneider *et al.* 2005). Recently the Alzheimer's Society led on a guidance document for the management of these symptoms (Ballard *et al.* 2009). This highlighted the importance of non-pharmacological intervention to prevent the onset of such symptoms, and 'watchful waiting' for their management, highlighting the fact that the duration of these symptoms can be short-lived and may resolve spontaneously. The focus on person-centred care for patients with dementia in the care home setting has been shown to reduce neuropsychiatric symptoms in a randomised control setting (Chenoweth *et al.* 2009).

Conditions associated with dementia and their treatment

The syndrome of dementia per se has the specific symptoms mentioned above. There are, however, due to the age of the at-risk population, a number of conditions that are closely associated with dementia. This means that, during the course of an individual's time living with dementia, their health care needs are likely to encompass the following conditions, which should therefore be thought of as an important part of the treatment spectrum for dementia.

Delirium

Delirium is an acute change in an individual's mental state and is characterised by fluctuations with time and reduced attention that develops over days or hours. The specific diagnostic criteria according to the American Psychiatric Association's *Diagnostic and Statistical Manual of Mental Disorders*, 4th edition (DSM-IV), are shown in Box 4.3 (American Psychiatric Association 2000).

Box 4.3 Delirium: DSM-IV essential diagnostic criteria

- *Disturbance of consciousness* (i.e. reduced clarity of awareness of the environment) with reduced ability to focus, sustain or shift attention.
- *Change in cognition* (e.g. memory deficit, disorientation, language disturbance and perceptual disturbance) that is not better accounted for by a pre-existing, established or evolving dementia.
- *Development over a short period of time* (usually hours to days) and disturbance *tends to fluctuate* during the course of the day.
- There is *evidence* from the history, physical examination or laboratory findings that the *disturbance is caused by the direct physiological consequences of a general medical condition.*

Delirium is common, affecting 15 per cent of all acute adult hospital admissions and 25 per cent of acute geriatric medicine patients. Seven per cent of people over the age of 65 will develop delirium each year. It can present in a variety of ways, including behavioural disturbance and a change in functional ability, that is, a decline in their ability to perform everyday activities. It is very important to recognise and treat delirium when it occurs, as it is associated with a high mortality rate: one in five patients with delirium will be dead within a month. It is often very distressing for the individual affected and it increases their length of hospital inpatient stay, as well as increasing the likelihood of going into care homes. The complexity of delirium associated with illness and the symptoms of dementia is illustrated in Box 4.4.

The case study in Box 4.4 demonstrates in practice the complex issues that patients present. It also highlights the atypical way that acute illness and symptoms of delirium and dementia can present in the elderly population.

Box 4.4 Delirium: a case study highlighting the importance of investigating and managing acute confusion

---

Mr W, an 87-year-old gentleman, was admitted to hospital with increasing confusion. On admission he was unable to give a consistent history and unfortunately at that time his family was not present. The doctors were unaware of any past medical history and Mr W stated that he was not taking any regular medications.

On examination there were no findings: all observations were within the normal parameters – chest was clear, heart sounded pure and there was nil to note on abdominal or neurological examinations. A full infection screen was carried out, urine dipstick was negative and all blood tests were normal. Cognitive testing (Abbreviated Mental Test – AMT) was carried out with a very poor result, scoring only 2 out of 10.

Mr W was admitted to a general medical ward. He became increasingly difficult to manage: having hallucinations, wandering and requiring one-to-one supervision. Subsequently, he was moved to a geriatric assessment ward, where he had a further assessment and was diagnosed with delirium.

On further investigation looking into the reason for his delirium, it was found that his blood count was low. An endoscopy (looking into the gullet for any sources of bleeding) was carried out, which found an oesophageal ulcer with active bleeding, and this was successfully treated. It was felt that Mr W had become delirious secondary to his acute bleed. Once treated, his delirium began to settle.

On discussion with his relatives it became apparent that his brother, whom he had previously lived with, had passed away two weeks prior to admission. This was a crucial finding to understand the reason for admission and also for future discharge planning. The discharge was complex but through the use of the multi-agency approach Mr W was able to return to the community with a care package in place to support him. He later returned to the medical memory clinic in order to get a formal assessment of his cognition.

The state of delirium is traditionally classified as hyperactive (e.g. with disturbed sleep pattern, wandering behaviour, hallucinations) or hypo-active (e.g. with drowsiness and reduced conscious level). Delirium is commonly associated with acute illness (in some cases relatively minor illness), but increasing evidence suggests that in vulnerable individuals (e.g. those with dementia) an impaired response to stress hormones in the brain may play an important part (MacLullich *et al.* 2008). Delirium generally explains the worsening in dementia symptoms that are perceived by caregivers when an individual with dementia is taken out of the familiar surroundings of their own home in an unplanned fashion (e.g. for acute hospital admission). In this instance the cerebral response to stress hormones generated in this frightening scenario along with the acute illness itself will be factors adding to the precipitation of delirium.

Co-morbidity/polypharmacy

With increasing age (the strongest risk factor for dementia) the number of non-curative (chronic) diseases (e.g. hypertension, diabetes, heart failure) encountered by an individual increases. This results in significant co-morbidity in the population with dementia. Polypharmacy results from the numerous medications required for the treatment of these additional conditions.

Chronic disease management in itself can have a significant bearing on cognitive function: poorly controlled diabetes can have a detrimental effect on cognitive function, or lead to worsening chronic obstructive pulmonary disease (COPD) or heart failure and resulting chronic hypoxia, resulting in impaired oxygen delivery to the brain and consequently impaired brain function. In the population of individuals with dementia, poorly controlled chronic disease can result in what appears to be progression of the dementia itself. Improvement in the management of that chronic disease can therefore be seen to improve the symptoms of dementia; that is, to be a crucial part of the treatment of dementia.

Polypharmacy is defined as 'use of medications that are not clinically indicated' (Fulton *et al.* 2005) or using 'more than a certain number of drugs, irrespective of the appropriateness of drug use' (Nguyen *et al.* 2006). With increasing numbers of medications prescribed, the number of possible adverse drug interactions increases significantly. On average, adverse drug reactions account for 3–13 per cent of all hospital admissions in the elderly population (Manesse *et al.* 2000), and in themselves can precipitate the onset of delirium (e.g. hyponatraemia secondary to diureticuse, digoxin toxicity, etc.).

The problems surrounding polypharmacy are often forgotten. Many of the elderly population are on multiple drugs for multiple co-morbidities. Many drugs can result in admission due to the adverse reactions that they may cause. For example, evidence has shown that pro-cholinergics can successfully slow down the progression of dementia by boosting the neurotransmitters in the brain. This means that *anti*-cholinergics, which are often used in the treatment of dizziness and incontinence, can actually mimic the symptoms of dementia.

This is only one example of the side-effects of drugs, and highlights the importance of reviewing medications on admission.

The cholinergic effect of some treatment often goes un-noted. The prescription of medication that has a cholinergic effect has been shown to be associated with decline in cognitive function and increased mortality (Fox *et al.* 2011). This follows, as Alzheimer's disease has been shown to be characterised by a reduction in the neurotransmitter acelylcholine in the brain. Medication that has an effect of reducing this neurotransmitter can therefore be seen as having the potential to induce the symptoms of Alzheimer's disease. The level of the anti-cholinergic effect produced by different medications has been studied and individual risk calculated for each drug treatment (the cholinergic index). Those medications with high scores include anti-psychotics, antihistamines, and gastrointestinal and urinary antispasmodics. Medication with a high cholinergic index can therefore potentially mimic a worsening of dementia in affected individuals. These drugs should therefore be avoided in dementia.

Frailty

Frailty is a description of reduction in an individual's physiological reserve to respond to declining function, usually associated with aging. Frailty has been elegantly described by Rockwood as an accumulation of deficits which result in increasing disability and reduced facility for independent living (Mitnitski *et al.* 2001). A useful clinical definition is that used by the Gwent Frailty Project in South Wales (Gwent Frailty Programme), implemented in April 2011; see Box 4.5.

Box 4.5 Frailty

Three simultaneous components:

- *Dependency:* chronic limitations on activities of daily living associated with functional/physical/social impairment.
- *Vulnerability:* an overall loss of physiological reserved and functional stability.
- *Co-morbidity:* multiple ongoing medical conditions.

The management of frailty is not generally seen in biomedical terms of 'treat and cure' but rather as identifying and managing each one of the individual deficits in order to re-establish increasing levels of independence. Many individuals with dementia also have frailty and the management of their well-being requires attention to details of the frailty syndrome along with the dementia in order to preserve independence and quality of life as far as possible.

Quantification of deficiencies within the frailty syndrome can be documented in instances where an older person's well-being is assessed using a 'comprehensive geriatric assessment' (CGA) approach. The term CGA was first developed by Rubenstein in 1991 (Rubenstein *et al.* 1991). He described it as 'a multidimensional interdisciplinary diagnostic process focussed on determining a frail elderly person's medical, psychological and functional capability in order to develop a coordinated and integrated plan for treatment and long-term follow-up'. The four principal parts are:

1. *Physical health:* geriatric medicine specific including assessing for sensory impairment, continence and gait.

2. *Functional ability:* looking at an individual's ability to perform activities of daily living and how this has changed over time.

3. *Cognitive and mental health:* screening for memory problems, delirium and depression.

4. *Socio-environmental:* living situation and support at home. Involves collateral history from family members or carers and information from social services input.

Older people admitted with acute illness to hospitals in NHS Fife, Scotland, have been assessed this way since 2009. Audit data from this assessment have shown that in addition to cognitive impairment (a salient symptom of dementia) a significant number have had loss of basic activities of daily living (functional ability), falls, and difficulty coping at home (see Table 4.3). Optimising each one of these impairments in addition to treating underlying acute medical problems is the mainstay of treatment and care in order to maintain independence and quality of life.

Table 4.3 Audit data from comprehensive geriatric assessments colelcted in Fife NHS hospitals, Scotland

	Mean age	Mean memory score (/10)	Mean change in functional ability (/6)	History of falls	Percentage reporting difficulties at home	Percentage with existing dementia
Memory impairment	83	4.5	1.3	34%	34	24
No memory impairment	78	9.3	0.9	20%	19	1

Conclusion

Advocates for the integration of health and social care have highlighted the proven benefits to outcomes of fully integrated services. Those with dementia and their carers, by virtue of their vulnerability and demographics, typify a group who will benefit from integration.

The integration required for those with dementia to maintain independent and meaningful lives is best understood when the individual with dementia is central to the integration. This 'whole system approach' also needs to incorporate families, carers, the community and the third sector, plus all aspects of health and social care. Those with dementia will rely on the contributions of everyone around them to maintain a good quality of life.

There are, however, still many barriers that hamper the process by which a person with dementia is treated and cared for. There is a need for the public perception of dementia to shift, so that the condition is neither feared nor stigmatised. It should be seen as a condition with viable options for treatment, with the real possibility of improved outcomes (particularly after early diagnosis).

The diagnostic gap is a major issue in the UK, and is at its worst in acute settings. There can be few other conditions where 60 per cent of the affected population remain undiagnosed – a near-scandalous circumstance in the case of dementia. Part of the responsibility for under-diagnosis sits with health care professionals. GPs, for example, tend to view dementia in the elderly as a characteristic of aging and make the assumption that diagnosis will not improve outcome (with consequent reluctance to refer). In the general hospital setting clinicians may view dementia as a mental health problem, and so basic assessment of the symptoms of dementia is omitted. Clearly reluctance, even fear, among families of those with the early symptoms of dementia will further limit opportunities for diagnosis. Social care professionals may well have extensive dealings with those with early symptoms, but have neither the training in, or access to, the diagnostic process.

The delivery of evidence-based treatment appears disjointed: the treatment of Alzheimer's disease is widely seen as the territory of mental health teams, while those with vascular brain disease may be treated by a stroke physician. Alongside this, the conditions associated with dementia are perceived as the responsibility of general practice or geriatric medicine.

The momentum to drive change and improvement for dementia is high. This enthusiasm should be harnessed in addressing the challenges identified in this chapter. The solutions lie in greater acceptance by all associated with dementia that multicomponent intervention addressing all of these domains is fundamental for sustained optimal treatment and care for all people with dementia.

References

Alzheimer Europe (2010) *European Collaboration on Dementia.* Available at www.alzheimer-europe.org/EN/Research/European-Collaboration-on-Dementia

Alzheimer Europe (2011) *National Dementia Plans.* Available at www.alzheimer-europe.org/EN/Policy-in-Practice2/National-Dementia-Plans

Alzheimer's Association (2009) *Alzheimer's Association Early Detection Alliance.* Available at www.alz.org/aeda/aeda.asp

Alzheimer's Disease International (2010) *World Alzheimer Report 2010: The Global Economic Impact of Dementia.* Available at www.alz.co.uk/research/files/WorldAlzheimerReport2010ExecutiveSummary.pdf

Alzheimer's Society (2002) *Younger People with Dementia.* Available at www.alzheimers.org.uk/ypwd) and http://alzheimers.org.uk/site/scripts/download_info.php?fileID=1058

Alzheimer's Society (2011a) *Mapping the Dementia Gap.* Available at http://alzheimers.org.uk/site/scripts/download_info.php?fileID=1058

Alzheimer's Society (2011b) *Optimising Treatment and Care for Behavioural and Psychological Symptoms of Dementia.* Available at http://alzheimers.org.uk/site/scripts/documents_info.php?documentID=1657

American Psychiatric Association (2000) *Diagnostic and Statistical Manual of Mental Disorders, 4th Edition (DSM-IV) Text Revision.* Washington, DC: American Psychiatric Association.

Ballard, C. *et al.* (2009) 'The dementia antipsychotic withdrawal trial (DART-AD): long-term follow-up of a randomised placebo-controlled trial.' *Lancet Neurology 8,* 2, 151–157.

Banerjee, S. *et al.* (2007) 'Improving the quality of care for mild to moderate dementia.' *International Journal of Geriatric Psychiatry 22,* 8, 782–788.

Birks, J. (2006) 'Cholinesterase inhibitors for Alzheimer's disease.' *Cochrane Database of Systematic Reviews,* Issue 1. Art. No.: CD005593. doi:10.1002/14651858.CD005593

Blendon, R.J. *et al.* (2011) 'Key findings from a five-country survey of public attitudes about Alzheimer's disease.' Poster presented at Alzheimer's Association International Conference, July 2011.

British Geriatrics Society (2010) *Dignity Campaign 2010.* Available at www.bgs.org.uk/campaigns/dignity2010.html

Chenoweth, L. *et al.* (2009) 'Caring for Aged Dementia Care Resident Study (CADRES) of person-centred care, dementia-care mapping, and usual care in dementia: a cluster-randomised trial.' *Lancet Neurology 8,* 4, 317–325.

Cohen, D. *et al.* (1990) 'Caring for relatives with Alzheimer's disease: the mental health risks to spouses, adult children, and other family caregivers.' *Behavior, Health, and Aging 1*, 3, 171–182.

Covinsky, K.E. *et al.* (2003) 'Patient and caregiver characteristics associated with depression in caregivers of patients with dementia.' *Journal of General Internal Medicine 18*, 12, 1006–1014.

Craig, D. *et al.* (2005) 'A cross-sectional study of neuropsychiatric symptoms in 435 patients with Alzheimer's disease.' *American Journal of Geriatric Psychiatry 13*, 6, 460–468.

DeKosky, S. (2003) 'Early intervention is key to successful management of Alzheimer disease.' *Alzheimer Disease and Associated Disorder 17*, S99–S104.

Dementia Rights (2009) *Charter of Rights for People with Dementia and their Carers in Scotland.* Available at www.dementiarights.org/charter-of-rights

Department of Health (2010) *Quality Outcomes for People with Dementia: Building on the Work of the National Dementia Strategy.* Available at www.dh.gov.uk/en/SocialCare/NationalDementiaStrategy/index.htm

Evans, D.A. (1996) 'The epidemiology of dementia and Alzheimer's disease: an evolving field.' *Journal of the American Geriatric Society 44*, 12, 1482–1483.

Fox, C. *et al.* (2011) 'Anticholinergic medication use and cognitive impairment in the older population: the medical research council cognitive function and ageing study.' *Journal of the American Geriatrics Society 59*, 8, 1477–1483.

Fulton, M.M. *et al.* (2005) 'Polypharmacy in the elderly: a literature review.' *Journal of the American Academy of Nurse Practitioners 17*, 123–132.

General Register Office for Scotland (2010) *Mid-2009 Population Estimates for Scotland.* Available at www.gro-scotland.gov.uk/statistics/theme/population/estimates/mid-year/2009/index.html

George, L.K. *et al.* (1986) 'Caregiver well-being: a multidimensional examination of family caregivers of demented adults.' *Gerontologist 26*, 253–259.

Gwent Frailty Programme (implemented April 2011). Available at www.gwentfrailty.torfaen.gov.uk

Heart Protection Study Collaborative Group (2002) 'MRC/BHF Heart Protection Study of cholesterol lowering with simvastatin in 20,536 high-risk individuals: a randomised placebo-controlled trial.' *Lancet 360*, 9326, 7–22.

Hofman, A. *et al.* (1991) 'The prevalence of dementia in Europe: a collaborative study of 1980–1990 findings.' EURODEM Prevalence Research Group. *International Journal of Epidemiology 20*, 3, 736–748.

Hyman, B.T. *et al.* (1984) 'Alzheimer's disease: cell-specific pathology isolates the hippocampal formation.' *Science 225*, 4667, 1168–1170.

Kiecolt-Glaser, J.K. *et al.* (1991) 'Spousal caregivers of dementia victims: longitudinal changes in immunity and health.' *Psychosomatic Medicine 53*, 4, 345–362.

King, A.C. *et al.* (1994) 'Ambulatory blood pressure and heart rate responses to the stress of work and caregiving in older women.' *Journal of Gerontology 49*, M239–245.

Kitwood, T. (1993) 'Person and process in dementia.' *International Journal of Geriatric Psychiatry 8*, 7, 541–545.

Kivipelto, M. *et al.* (2001) 'Midlife vascular risk factors and Alzheimer's disease in later life: longitudinal, population based study.' *British Medical Journal 322*, 1447.

MacLullich, A.M.J. *et al.* (2008) 'Unravelling the pathophysiology of delirium: a focus on the role of aberrant stress responses.' *Journal of Psychosomatic Research 65*, 3, 229–238.

Mannesse, C.K. *et al.* (2000) 'Contribution of adverse drug reactions to hospital admission of older patients.' *Age and Ageing 29*, 35–39.

Mitnitski, A.B. *et al.* (2001) 'Accumulation of deficits as a proxy measure of aging.' *Scientific World Journal 1*, 323–336.

Mittelman, M.S. (2007) 'Preserving health of Alzheimer caregivers: impact of a spouse caregiver intervention.' *American Journal of Geriatric Psychiatry 15*, 9, 780–789.

Moniz-Cook, E. *et al.* (1998) 'A preliminary study of the effects of early intervention with people with dementia and their families in a memory clinic.' *Aging and Mental Health 2*, 3, 199–213.

Mulsant, B. *et al.* (2003) 'Serum anticholinergic activity in a community-based sample of older adults: relationship with cognitive performance.' *Archives of General Psychiatry 60*, 198–203.

Nair, B.K. *et al.* (2011) 'The effect of Baroque music on behavioural disturbances in patients with dementia.' *Australasian Journal on Ageing 30*, 1, 11–15.

National Care Forum (2007) *Promoting Quality Care through the Not-For-Profit Sector.* Available at www.nationalcareforum.org.uk/content/Key principles of person-centred dementia care.pdf

Nguyen, J.K. *et al.* (2006) 'Polypharmacy as a risk factor for adverse drug reactions in geriatric nursing home residents.' *The American Journal of Geriatric Pharmacotherapy 4*, 1, 36–41.

NICE (2011a) *Vascular Disease – Clopidogrel and Dipyridamol.* Available at http://guidance.nice.org.uk/TA210

NICE (2011b) *Technology Appraisals (TA217). Alzheimer Disease – Donepezil, Galantamine, Rivastigmin and Memantine.* Available at http://guidance.nice.org.uk/TA2/7

Ory, M.G. *et al.* (1999) 'Prevalence and impact of caregiving: a detailed comparison between dementia and nondementia caregivers.' *Gerontologist 39*, 2, 177–186.

Pinquart, M. (2003) 'Differences between caregivers and noncaregivers in psychological health and physical health: a meta-analysis.' *Psychology and Aging 18*, 2, 250–267.

PROGRESS Collaborative Group (2001) 'Randomised trial of a perindopril-based blood-pressure-lowering regimen among 6,105 individuals with previous stroke or transient ischaemic attack.' *Lancet 358*, 1033–1041.

Reisberg, B. *et al.* for the Memantine Study Group (2003) 'Memantine in Moderate-to-Severe Alzheimer's Disease.' *New England Journal of Medicine 348*, 1333–1341.

Rubenstein, L.Z. *et al.* (1991) 'Impacts of geriatric evaluation and management programs on defined outcomes: overview of the evidence.' *Journal of the American Geriatrics Society 39*, 8S–16S; discussion 17S–18S.

Sampson, E. *et al.* (2009) 'Dementia in the acute hospital: prospective cohort study of prevalence and mortality.' *British Journal of Psychiatry 195*, 61–66.

Schneider, L.S. *et al.* (2005) 'Risk of death with atypical antipsychotic drug treatment for dementia: meta-analysis of randomized placebo-controlled trials.' *Journal of the American Medical Association 294*, 15, 1934–1943.

Schulz, R. *et al.* (1995) 'Psychiatric and physical morbidity effects of dementia caregiving: Prevalence, correlates, and causes.' *Gerontologist 35*, 6, 771–791.

Schulz, R. *et al.* (1999) 'Caregiving as a risk factor for mortality: the Caregiver Health Effects Study.' *Journal of the American Medical Association 282*, 2215–2219.

Stroke Prevention in Atrial Fibrillation investigators (1991) 'Stroke Prevention in Atrial Fibrillation Study: final results.' *Circulation 84*, 527–539.

Stroke Prevention in Atrial Fibrillation investigators (1994) 'Warfarin versus aspirin for prevention of thromboembolism in atrial fibrillation: Stroke Prevention in Atrial Fibrillation II Study.' *Lancet 343*, 8899, 687–691.

Stroke Prevention in Atrial Fibrillation investigators (1996) 'Adjusted-dose warfarin versus low-intensity, fixed-dose warfarin plus aspirin for high-risk patients with atrial fibrillation: Stroke Prevention in Atrial Fibrillation III randomised clinical trial.' *Lancet 348*, 9028, 633–638.

Williamson, G.M. *et al.* (1993) 'Coping with specific stressors in Alzheimer's disease caregiving.' *Gerontologist 33*, 6, 747–755.

Part II

POLICY

DEVELOPMENT

Chapter 5

Policy to Enable People to Live Well with Dementia

DEVELOPMENT OF THE NATIONAL DEMENTIA STRATEGY FOR ENGLAND

Sube Banerjee

Introduction

Dementia is one of the greatest societal policy challenges that we face. The profound negative impacts of dementia on people with dementia themselves and their families, and in terms of health and social service use, are not in doubt. Powerful misconceptions exist concerning dementia, including: it being a normal part of aging; that there is nothing that can be done to help; and that it is better not to know. These have resulted in a situation where dementia has not been a priority for health policy makers and commissions.

The direct result of this is that the large majority of people with dementia and their family carers do not benefit from the positive intervention and support that can promote well-being and prevent crises for all involved. At times it can seem that services have been designed to result in the avoidance of diagnosis and the consequent denial of care. In the UK only about a third of people with dementia receive a diagnosis of dementia. When they do, it is usually late in the disorder, often at a time of crisis when it is too late to prevent the harm that has been caused to the person with dementia and their family (National Audit Office [NAO] 2007). This chapter focuses on the development and the content of the English National Dementia Strategy which attempts to address this.

Policy is site-specific; it only functions in the circumstances and jurisdiction that it was developed to serve. So the National Dementia Strategy described here applies only in England and not in the other parts of the United Kingdom: Scotland, Wales and Northern Ireland. Responsibility for health policy in each of these countries is devolved to the parliaments and assemblies that govern these countries. They would no more accept English policy (no matter what its content) than they would support an English soccer team against their own country. It is therefore a well-observed finding that near neighbours, similar systems of care notwithstanding, will require separate strategy and policy development if it is to be owned by that jurisdiction. For a policy or strategy to be successful it needs local ownership, so, just as with politics, all successful policy and strategy is local.

Policy development

Strategy and policy evolves and, as the evidence base has grown, so the last decade has seen a growing acknowledgement and understanding of the challenge posed by dementia and the need for service improvement. To illustrate the building blocks, details of relevant UK reports and policy include:

- *Forget Me Not: Mental Health Services for Older People* (Audit Commission 2000). Key findings included:

    - Only a half of general practitioners (GPs) believed it important to look actively for signs of dementia and to make an early diagnosis.

    - Less than half of GPs felt that they had received sufficient training in how to diagnose dementia.

    - A lack of clear information, counselling, advocacy and support for people with dementia and their family carers.

    - An insufficient supply of specialist home care.

    - Poor quality assessment and treatment, with little joint health and social care planning and working.

    Little improvement was found when reviewing change two years later (Audit Commission 2002).

- *The National Service Framework for Older People* (Department of Health [DH] 2001) included a chapter on mental health and older people, including a consideration of dementia, advocating:

    - early diagnosis and intervention

    - that the National Health Service (NHS) and local authorities should review arrangements for health promotion, early detection and diagnosis, assessment, care and treatment planning, and access to specialist services

    - the provision of 'integrated' and 'comprehensive' services.

Reviewing progress, this appears to have had little positive impact on services for people with dementia and their families (Banerjee, Graham and Gurland 2010).

- *Everybody's Business. Integrated Mental Health Services for Older Adults: A Service Development Guide* (Care Services Improvement Partnership 2005). This set out the essentials for a service that works for older people's mental health, including:

  ○ memory assessment services to enable early diagnosis of dementia for all

  ○ integrated community mental health teams whose role includes the management of people with dementia with complex behavioural and psychological symptoms.

  Little effect has been seen from this, since there were no levers to mandate such service provision.

- *Dementia: Supporting People with Dementia and their Carers in Health and Social Care. A Joint Clinical Guideline on the Management of Dementia* (National Institute for Health and Clinical Excellence, and Social Care Institute of Excellence 2006). Key recommendations included:

  ○ integrated working across all agencies

  ○ memory assessment services as a point of referral for diagnosis of dementia

  ○ assessment, support and treatment (where needed) for carers

  ○ assessment and treatment of non-cognitive symptoms and behaviour that challenges

  ○ dementia care training for all staff working with older people

  ○ improvement of care for people with dementia in general hospitals.

  This is a useful, if unprioritised, list of things that might be done but are generally not done. Publication of this guideline did not prompt change in services but showed what might be done.

- *The Dementia UK Report* (Knapp *et al.* 2007), published by the Alzheimer's Society. The report's key findings included:

  ○ the number of people with dementia in the UK in 2007 – 700,000

  ○ the projected number of people with dementia in the UK – doubling in 30 years to 1.4 million

- the costs of dementia – £17 billion per year
- low level of diagnosis and management of dementia in the UK
- high variation in activity between areas in the UK
- the recommendation that dementia should be made an explicit national health and social care priority
- the need to improve the quality of services provided for people with dementia and their carers.

This report has had a positive impact in terms of the Government accepting the figures and the need to do something to improve care and, along with the next two reports, it has formed the basis for making dementia a priority and developing national policy.

- *Improving Services and Support for People with Dementia* (NAO 2007). This report by the external auditors of UK governmental spending was profoundly critical of the quality of care received by people with dementia and their families. Its findings included:

  - The size and availability of specialist community mental health teams was extremely variable.
  - The confidence of GPs in spotting the symptoms of dementia was poor and lower than it had been in 2000 (down to a third).
  - Deficiencies in carer support.
  - Services are not currently delivering value for money to taxpayers or people with dementia and their families.
  - Too few people are being diagnosed or being diagnosed early enough.
  - Early diagnosis and intervention is needed to improve quality of life.
  - Services in the community, care homes and at the end of life are not delivering consistently or cost-effectively against the objective of supporting people to live independently as long as possible in the place of their choosing.
  - There is need for a 'spend to save' approach, with upfront investment in services, for early diagnosis and intervention and improved specialist services and community services, and in general hospitals, resulting in long-term cost savings from prevention of transition into care homes and decreased length of hospital stay.

This report required a high-level response from Government and very much helped in the prioritisation of dementia, forming part of the rationale for the National Dementia Strategy.

- *Improving Services and Support for People with Dementia* (Public Accounts Committee [PAC] 2008). NAO reports are followed up by the PAC, which is the senior committee of the House of Commons and which holds to account by interrogation the heads of the civil service responsible for government spending, in this case the DH. At the committee's public hearing on 15 October 2007 the NHS Chief Executive and other senior policy makers from the DH were questioned on the NAO's criticisms. The PAC's subsequent recommendations included:

  o dementia to be made a high priority for the NHS and social care

  o the need for explicit national ownership and leadership

  o early diagnosis

  o improving public attitudes and understanding

  o coordinated care

  o all improvements to benefit carers too

  o improvements in care in care homes

  o improvements in care in general hospitals.

The Government's response to this report was to accept virtually all the conclusions and recommendations of the committee, assuring the committee that their findings would be fully addressed in a new National Dementia Strategy. In preparation for this there was a one-year programme to develop a National Dementia Strategy and implementation plan.

Developing the National Dementia Strategy

From the start it was decided that the strategy should be designed to address the needs of all people with dementia, no matter of what type, age, ethnic origin or social status. A second important primary decision was to enter into as full a consultation as possible. An External Reference Group (ERG) was convened and chaired independently of the DH by the Chief Executive of the UK Alzheimer's Society. A further strength was that the many reports that over the years had identified flaws in the system meant that there was a consensus as to the areas needing attention from the start. The overall structure developed as a framework for this work stood up well in the development process. It was structured along three themes:

1. Improving public and professional attitudes and understanding of dementia.

2. Early diagnosis and intervention for all.

3. Good quality care and support at all stages, from diagnosis through to the end of life.

Three ERG sub-groups worked on these themes generating a comprehensive report on improving dementia care which informed but did not determine the development of the strategy. The development included two waves of formal external consultation organised jointly by the DH and the Alzheimer's Society. The first, completed prior to developing the consultation document, involved a nationwide listening and engagement exercise where more than 3000 people were able to contribute to and engage with developing the strategy. The Alzheimer's Society ran similar events especially for people with dementia and carers and distributed questionnaires, both through the Society's branches and online. Feedback from all these sources was reviewed to ensure that all views were captured.

A consultation document containing draft proposals was then generated by a DH strategy working group co-chaired by a senior social services leader and a senior dementia specialist from a health background (DH 2008). This acknowledged the need for joint and integrative approaches throughout. In the second phase DH held a formal public consultation exercise on the draft proposals for the strategy, receiving over 600 written responses from individuals, including those with dementia and their carers, and a wide range of professional and other stakeholder groups. These responses were analysed and informed the development of the final strategy. In addition 53 further regional consultation events were held; over 4000 individuals attended these meetings. Meetings covered the whole country including rural and urban areas; again specific groups were targeted to ensure that the views of diverse populations had been included in the development of the strategy, such as: people with dementia themselves, people with learning disabilities, people from minority ethnic groups, and older people in prisons and remote and island communities. Officials from DH attended all these meetings as well as other dementia-related conferences and meetings across the country to publicise the consultation and gather feedback.

This process was time-consuming and labour-intensive but of value, since the inclusiveness and comprehensiveness of the development and consultation process for such a strategy lends it both validity and power when moving towards implementation.

The National Dementia Strategy – Living Well with Dementia

Finally, the National Dementia Strategy (NDS) was published in February 2009 (DH 2009). The 17 interlinked objectives of the final strategy are presented in Box 5.1, along with the summary paragraphs used in the strategy. It presents a comprehensive critical analysis of the current systems of providing health and social care for people with dementia and their carers. The objectives are not in order of priority but according to the narrative of the strategy, which is based on a notional pathway through care.

Box 5.1 Objectives of the National Dementia Strategy

Objective 1: Improving public and professional awareness and understanding of dementia. Public and professional awareness and understanding of dementia to be improved and the stigma associated with it addressed. This should inform individuals of the benefits of timely diagnosis and care, promote the prevention of dementia, and reduce social exclusion and discrimination. It should encourage behaviour change in terms of appropriate help-seeking and help provision.

Objective 2: Good-quality early diagnosis and intervention for all. All people with dementia to have access to a pathway of care that delivers: a rapid and competent specialist assessment; an accurate diagnosis, sensitively communicated to the person with dementia and their carers; and treatment, care and support provided as needed following diagnosis. The system needs to have the capacity to see all new cases of dementia in the area.

Objective 3: Good-quality information for those with diagnosed dementia and their carers. Providing people with dementia and their carers with good-quality information on the illness and on the services available, both at diagnosis and throughout the course of their care.

Objective 4: Enabling easy access to care, support and advice following diagnosis. A dementia adviser to facilitate easy access to appropriate care, support and advice for those diagnosed with dementia and their carers.

Objective 5: Development of structured peer support and learning networks. The establishment and maintenance of such networks will provide direct local peer support for people with dementia and their carers. It will also enable people with dementia and their carers to take an active role in the development and prioritisation of local services.

Objective 6: Improved community personal support services. Provision of an appropriate range of services to support people with dementia living at home and their carers. Access to flexible and reliable services, ranging from early intervention to specialist home care services, which are responsive to the personal needs and preferences of each individual and take account of their broader family circumstances. Accessible to people living alone or with carers, and people who pay for their care privately, through personal budgets or through local authority-arranged services.

Objective 7: Implementing the Carers' Strategy. Family carers are the most important resource available for people with dementia. Active work is needed to ensure that the provisions of the Carers' Strategy are available for carers of people with dementia. Carers have a right to an assessment of their needs and can be supported through an agreed plan to support the important role they play in the care of the person with dementia. This will include good-quality, personalised breaks. Action should also be taken to strengthen support for children who are in caring roles, ensuring that their particular needs as children are protected.

Objective 8: Improved quality of care for people with dementia in general hospitals. Identifying leadership for dementia in general hospitals, defining the care pathway for dementia there and the commissioning of specialist liaison older people's mental health teams to work in general hospitals.

Objective 9: Improved intermediate care for people with dementia. Intermediate care which is accessible to people with dementia and which meets their needs.

Objective 10: Considering the potential for housing support, housing-related services and telecare to support people with dementia and their carers. The needs of people with dementia and their carers should be included in the development of housing options, assistive technology and telecare. As evidence emerges, commissioners should consider the provision of options to prolong independent living and delay reliance on more intensive services.

Objective 11: Living well with dementia in care homes. Improved quality of care for people with dementia in care homes by the development of explicit leadership for dementia within care homes, defining the care pathway there, the commissioning of specialist in-reach services from community mental health teams, and through inspection regimes.

Objective 12: Improved end of life care for people with dementia. People with dementia and their carers to be involved in planning end of life care which recognises the principles outlined in the Department of Health

End of Life Care Strategy. Local work on the End of Life Care Strategy to consider dementia.

Objective 13: An informed and effective workforce for people with dementia. Health and social care staff involved in the care of people who may have dementia to have the necessary skills to provide the best quality of care in the roles and settings where they work. To be achieved by effective basic training and continuous professional and vocational development in dementia.

Objective 14: A joint commissioning strategy for dementia. Local commissioning and planning mechanisms to be established to determine the services needed for people with dementia and their carers, and how best to meet these needs. These commissioning plans should be informed by the World Class Commissioning guidance for dementia developed to support this Strategy.

Objective 15: Improved assessment and regulation of health and care services and of how systems are working for people with dementia and their carers. Inspection regimes for care homes and other services that better assure the quality of dementia care provided.

Objective 16: A clear picture of research evidence and needs. Evidence to be available on the existing research base on dementia in the UK and gaps that need to be filled.

Objective 17: Effective national and regional support for implementation of the Strategy. Appropriate national and regional support to be available to advise and assist local implementation of the Strategy. Good-quality information to be available on the development of dementia services, including information from evaluations and demonstrator sites.

Implementation

It would be all too easy to believe that, with the formulation of a strategy, the work is done. However, the final phase is implementation, and that is a profound challenge. We are approaching the halfway mark in the proposed five-year plan and the question has to be: What has been achieved?

Each element of the NDS requires operationalisation in order to deliver the objective. Systems, therefore, needed to be put in place to work out exactly how each can be achieved, and progress has been patchy.

The first real test of the NDS was the change of government in the UK in 2010. Only a year in, could the NDS survive? Would it be downgraded in the rush to achieve localism and to reduce the number of top-down imperatives from the centre? This can be seen as the first real test of the strength of the document and the plan. In 2010 it was striking that dementia had been mentioned in all three main party manifestos for the very first time. It is a positive sign of the potential survivability of a policy area if the three main parties have all identified the political and health/social capital that may be gained by being associated with and delivering on an issue. President Sarkozy's championing of Alzheimer's disease during his candidacy for the French presidency and his delivery of the French *Plan Alzheimer* in his first year in power is a clear example of the emerging political value of Alzheimer's disease.

With the emergence of the coalition, dementia was only mentioned in the coalition agreement in terms of the prioritisation of 'dementia research within the health research and development budget'. However, the appointment of a minister (Paul Burstow, Lib Dem) with a strong track record in championing improvements in dementia care was potentially a positive step for people with dementia. The new government reviewed the NHS Operating Framework they had inherited and signalled continued movement towards local priority and decision-making. This meant a movement away from things generated nationally, such as the NDS. However, the document *Revision to the Operating Framework for the NHS in England 2010/11* contained positive news for dementia. In it dementia was one of only two new specific priorities:

> During the recent sign-off of SHAs plans, two areas stood out as not being given sufficient emphasis. The first is ensuring that military veterans receive appropriate treatment... The second area is dementia. NHS organisations should be working with partners on implementing the National Dementia Strategy. People with dementia and their families need information that helps them understand their local services, and the level of quality and outcomes that they can expect. PCTs [primary care trusts] and their partners should publish how they are implementing the National Dementia Strategy to increase local accountability for prioritisation. (DH 2010a)

Following this the Department of Health issued the document *Quality Outcomes for People with Dementia: Building on the Outcomes of the National Dementia Strategy*. In this they stated:

> There are four priority areas for the Department of Health's policy development work during 2010/11 to support local delivery of the Strategy. These areas provide a real focus on activities that are likely to have the greatest impact on improving quality outcomes for people with dementia and their carers. It is important to emphasise however that the priorities are enablers for local delivery of the Strategy in full, across all

17 objectives, as well as the work to implement the recommendations of the report in to the over-prescribing of antipsychotic medicines to people with dementia.

The four priority areas are:

- Good quality early diagnosis and intervention for all – Two thirds of people with dementia never receive a diagnosis; the UK is in the bottom third of countries in Europe for diagnosis and treatment of people with dementia; only a third of GPs feel they have adequate training in diagnosis of dementia.

- Improved quality of care in general hospitals – 40% of people in hospital have dementia; the excess cost is estimated to be £6m per annum in the average General Hospital; co-morbidity with general medical conditions is high, people with dementia stay longer in hospital.

- Living well with dementia in care homes – Two thirds of people in care homes have dementia; dependency is increasing; over half are poorly occupied; behavioural disturbances are highly prevalent and are often treated with antipsychotic drugs.

- Reduced use of antipsychotic medication – There are an estimated 180,000 people with dementia on antipsychotic drugs. In only about one third of these cases are the drugs having a beneficial effect and there are 1800 excess deaths per year as a result of their prescription.

(DH 2010b, pp.9–10)

This represents a reasonable restating of the priorities of the NDS with a reformulation into four main areas for action. All that is left is the action itself and evidence that it is being taken.

Soon afterwards the Secretary of State announced the development of a 'Commissioning Pack' for dementia. This is supposed to be a tool to help commissioners improve the quality of services for patients, through clearly defined outcomes that help drive efficiency by reducing unwarranted variation in services. Each pack is to contain: a set of tailored guidance, templates, tools and information to assist commissioners in commissioning health care services from existing providers, or for use in new procurements, and an evidence-based service specification which ensures that patients are placed at the forefront of the service and are central to decisions about their care.

This is supposed to be a nudge to new commissioners rather than an order, so the specification is non-mandatory and can be adapted to reflect local needs and, once agreed with the provider, should inform part of a renegotiated contract or form the relevant section of the NHS standard contract. The rationale is that by bringing together the clinical, financial and commercial aspects of commissioning in one place, the packs simplify processes and minimise bureaucracy. The dementia pack was published in summer 2011. The impact on commissioning decisions in the real NHS will need to be observed.

The area where there has been most noise has probably been the use of antipsychotic drugs for people with dementia. In the NDS this issue was included in the care home objective (Objective 11). This was acknowledged as such a priority that the Minister commissioned a review and the formulation of an action plan to run alongside the development of the NDS. This was completed and published in November 2009 (Banerjee 2009), and the summary recommendations presented in Box 5.2 provide an illustration of the detail of the secondary work needed to deliver the NDS. The order does not indicate priority (the recommendations should all be considered to have equal priority); neither does it indicate the sequence for their implementation.

Box 5.2 Recommendations to deliver improvements in the use of antipsychotic medication for people with dementia

Recommendation 1: Reducing the use of antipsychotic drugs for people with dementia and assuring good practice when they are needed should be made a clinical governance priority across the NHS. Using their existing clinical governance structures, Medical Directors (or their equivalent) in all primary care trusts, all mental health trusts and all acute trusts should review their level of risk in this area and ensure that systems and services are put in place to ensure good practice in the initiation, maintenance and cessation of these drugs for people with dementia.

Recommendation 2: National leadership for reducing the level of prescription of antipsychotic medication for people with dementia should be provided by the National Clinical Director for Dementia, working with local and national services. He or she should report on a six-monthly basis to the Minister of State for Care Services on progress against the recommendations in this review.

Recommendation 3: The National Clinical Director for Dementia should develop, with national and local clinical audit structures and leads, an audit to generate data on the use of antipsychotic medication for people with dementia in each primary care trust in England. This audit should be completed as soon as possible following the publication of this report, generating baseline data across England. It should be repeated one, two and three years later to gauge progress.

Recommendation 4: People with dementia should receive antipsychotic medication only when they really need it. To achieve this, there is a need for clear, realistic but ambitious goals to be agreed for the reduction of the use of antipsychotics for people with dementia. Explicit goals for the size and speed of this reduction in the use of antipsychotics in dementia, and improvement in their use where needed, should be agreed and published locally following the completion of the baseline audit. These goals should be reviewed yearly at primary care trust, regional and national level, with information published yearly on progress towards them at each level.

Recommendation 5: There is a need for further research to be completed, including work assessing the clinical and cost effectiveness of non-pharmacological methods of treating behavioural problems in dementia and of other pharmacological approaches as an alternative to antipsychotic medication. The National Institute for Health Research and the Medical Research Council should work to develop programmes of work in this area.

Recommendation 6: The Royal Colleges of General Practitioners, Psychiatrists, Nursing and Physicians should develop a curriculum for the development of appropriate skills for GPs and others working in care homes, to equip them for their role in the management of the complexity, co-morbidity and severity of mental and physical disorder in those now residing in care homes. This should be available as part of continuing professional development.

Recommendation 7: There is a need to develop a curriculum for the development of appropriate skills for care home staff in the non-pharmacological treatment of behavioural disorder in dementia, including the deployment of specific therapies with positive impact. Senior staff in care homes should have these skills and the ability to transfer them to other staff members in care homes. A national vocational qualification in dementia care should be developed for those working with people with dementia.

Recommendation 8: Each primary care trust should commission from local specialist older people's mental health services an in-reach service that supports primary care in its work in care homes. This extension of service needs the capacity to work routinely in all care homes where there may be people with dementia. They may be aided by regular pharmacist input into homes. This is a core recommendation of this report and it requires new capacity to be commissioned by primary care trusts in order that the other recommendations can be met.

Recommendation 9: The Care Quality Commission should consider using rates of prescription of antipsychotic medication for people with dementia, adherence to good practice guidelines, the availability of skills in non-pharmacological management of behavioural and psychological symptoms in dementia and the establishment of care home in-reach from specialist mental health services as markers of the quality of care provided by care homes. These data should be available by analysis of local audit data and commissioning decisions.

Recommendation 10: The Improving Access to Psychological Therapies programme should ensure that resources are made available for the delivery of therapies to people with dementia and their carers. Information and support should be available to carers to give them the skills needed to spot behavioural problems quickly, to seek help early and to deploy elements of non-pharmacological care themselves in the home.

Recommendation 11: Specialist older people's mental health services and GPs should meet in order to plan how to address the issue of people with dementia in their own homes who are on antipsychotic medication. Using practice and patient-level data from the completed audits on the use of these medications, they should agree how best to review and manage existing cases and how to ensure that future use follows best practice in terms of initiation, dose minimisation and cessation.

Soon after the change in government, 'Panorama', an investigative reporting television programme, aired a film on this subject, following up earlier work. It made clear the potential risks of these medications and questioned the willingness of the Government to act. The Minister appeared on the programme and promised that the target set in the report (a reduction to a third of current use) would be met within a year. This is a bold commitment and one which was more ambitious than that set out in the report (a three-year period for the reduction). It is unclear whether this target has been met to date (2011). The use of central government levers in the form of the commissioning packs and the quality outcomes, discussed above, which came after this television appearance, can be understood in this context.

However, the success or failure of any element of the NDS, and the NDS as a whole, falls to NHS and social care systems that are in turmoil from reorganisation and from the effects of budgetary restrictions following the credit crunch. In England, decisions on what to invest in for health currently lie at a local level, with around 150 PCTs. Convincing these commissioners that investing in dementia services is 'worth it' would be a complex marathon in itself. But to do so at a time when these PCTs are to be dismantled and a set of primary care commissioners put in their place, with major political questions about the role of the private sector, is more of an obstacle race where no-one knows the length of the race or which way around the track they should run.

What success requires is leadership at a local level as well as at a national level. The plan was for local implementation with regional support and national coordination in an iterative programme with staged introduction of the 17 elements of the strategy across the country in a logical order. Now the regional layers are being abolished and the central and local elements subject to massive reorganisation. The reality is that with the publication of the National Dementia Strategy the work to truly change things for people with dementia and their carers is only just beginning, and halfway through we have major decisions still to make and the way ahead is not clear.

In terms of the implementation to date (2011) there are positive signs. As said, at the time of writing this we are about halfway through the strategy's five-year implementation period. To delineate exactly what has happened to date is beyond the scope of this chapter, but some comment is needed. There are positive signs. It is excellent that the Department of Health, after some equivocation, has appointed a National Clinical Director for Dementia, and the post holder, Professor Alistair Burns, is doing an excellent job in what are trying times. It is positive that the profile of dementia continues to grow, with campaigns funded by the Government and run in conjunction with the Alzheimer's Society starting to change public attitudes and opinion. It is good that commissioning guides for dementia have been developed and that it is on the agenda of the NHS Commissioning Board. The brave testimony of people like Sir Terry Prachett, who is someone who has dementia but is well enough to be knighted and to make entertaining programmes about dementia as well as continuing to write, challenges stereotypes of dementia as a state of total dependency. With these changes comes destigmatisation of dementia.

The formation of the Dementia Alliance and their joint commitment to driving down the prescription of antipsychotic drugs in dementia is positive (see www.dementiaaction.org.uk). It is positive that all over the country there are empowered clinicians making the case for improved services, and informed and interested commissioners making the decisions that will enable them to do so. All these people are helping to make a difference and to make the vision of the strategy come to life. However, for every success we do not know how many areas are going backwards or staying still. There is a major lack of good quality data with which to gauge the success and extent of implementation of the strategy. Policy makers and clinicians need data to see where things are and to determine what else needs to be done. This was identified in the strategy and it is unhelpful that we cannot know how things are progressing from year to year. Such data would in no way diminish the ability of local areas to make local decisions and set local priorities; it would simply allow all to know what has been decided and done.

What makes success likely in the end is that the case is so clear, and so are the components. Full implementation of the strategy was always likely to be the work of 15 years rather than five. We know that early diagnosis, effective intervention and support from diagnosis through the course of the illness can enable people to live well with dementia. We also know that improving health and social care outcomes in dementia in the short and medium term can have significant benefits for society, both now and in the future. One of the major threats to developed economies is the cost of long-term care. This is very largely made up of the costs of dementia care. Good quality dementia care is the solution to the problem of long-term care funding, not a problem in itself. Doing care well in dementia means doing it early; this is cheaper and brings better quality than doing it late with higher costs and lower quality. Using arguments such as this, we can succeed in implementing the NDS, but as the programme enters its second half, the timescale for delivery remains unclear.

References

Audit Commission (2000) *Forget Me Not: Mental Health Services for Older People.* London: Audit Commission.

Audit Commission (2002) *Forget Me Not 2002: Developing Mental Health Services for Older People in England.* London: Audit Commission.

Banerjee, S. (2009) *The Use of Antipsychotic Medication for People with Dementia: Time for Action.* A report for the Minister of State for Care Services. London: Department of Health.

Banerjee, S., Willis, R., Graham, N. and Gurland, B. (2010) 'ADI-QOL: a cross-national population-level framework for assessing the quality of life impacts of services and policies for people with dementia and their family carers.' *International Journal of Geriatric Psychiatry 25,* 3, 249–257.

Care Services Improvement Partnership (2005) *Everybody's Business.* Leeds: Care Services Improvement Partnership.

Department of Health (2001) *National Service Framework for Older People.* London: Department of Health.

Department of Health (2008) *Transforming the Quality of Dementia Care – Consultation on a National Dementia Strategy.* London: Department of Health.

Department of Health (2009) *Living Well with Dementia: A National Dementia Strategy.* London: Department of Health.

Department of Health (2010a) *Revision to the Operating Framework for the NHS in England 2010/11.* London: Department of Health.

Department of Health (2010b) *Quality Outcomes for People with Dementia: Building on the Outcomes of the National Dementia Strategy.* London: Department of Health.

Knapp, M., Prince, M., Albanese, E., Banerjee, S. *et al.* (2007) *Dementia UK.* London: The Alzheimer's Society.

National Audit Office (2007) *Improving Services and Support for People with Dementia.* London: National Audit Office.

National Institute for Health and Clinical Excellence, and Social Care Institute of Excellence (2006) *Dementia: Supporting People with Dementia and their Carers in Health and Social Care.* London: National Collaborating Centre for Mental Health.

Public Accounts Committee (2008) *Improving Services and Support for People with Dementia.* London: The Stationery Office.

Chapter 6

Three Alzheimer Plans in France (2008–2012)

Marie-Jo Guisset-Martinez

Introduction

This chapter will examine the different steps in public policy relating to Alzheimer's disease in France since 2001. Three plans for Alzheimer's disease and other dementias that drive the agenda in France were produced, in 2001–2004, 2004–2007 and 2008. This chapter will present analysis of the evolutions of dementia policy in terms of images; health and social care; governance and implementation processes; financing; and last but not least, the impact of the three plans on the lives of people with Alzheimer's disease. A brief overview of the two earlier plans is followed by a detailed presentation of the ongoing plan. Finally the main results will be presented along with analysis of the barriers to successful implementation over the first three years of the current plan. According to the existing epidemiological studies the estimation of the number of people with dementia in France is more than 800,000 (Reynish *et al.* 2009). Among them, 450,000 are within a health care pathway (Table Ronde de Monsieur le Président de la République 2011).

France: a ten-year strategy on dementia

The first two plans

A first national report (Girard and Canestri 2000) commissioned by the public authorities (ministers in charge of Health Solidarity and Elderly) was established in September 2000, by Professor Jean François Girard. This identified the stigma attached to dementia in French society and recommended development of a dedicated national strategy, as had been done previously for AIDS. Girard's report considered that any improvement concerning this 'emblematic disease' will benefit all older people, as they also suffer from stigma due to their age. The report identified four major problems to meet the needs of persons with dementia and their families: problems concerning the diagnosis; lack of provisions and services; inadequate coordination between the different providers in the health and care field; and the difficult issue of information for the public. Following Girard's report recommendations in October 2001 the French Ministry of Health adopted an initial 'Programme for people suffering from Alzheimer's and related diseases' (Alzheimer Grande Cause Nationale 2007). This plan aims to fill some of the gaps identified: diagnosis, care interventions, help and support for family carers, respect and dignity of people with dementia, and research.

The priorities of the 2001–2004 plan were:

- implementing a national network of memory consultants to facilitate access to a reliable diagnosis

- encouraging the creation of day care centres which were at that time an exceptional provision

- improving the quality of residential care settings to meet the needs of people with cognitive impairments.

Due to the perceived importance of dignity for people with dementia, it was decided to launch regional Round Tables coordinated by France Alzheimer, the French family caregivers association, to raise awareness of ethical issues.

In September 2004 a second three-year Alzheimer plan was launched to complete and improve what had been initiated during the first one. On the one hand, family organizations and representatives of professional bodies express their satisfaction about this next step, showing the political will to continue considering dementia as a national priority. On the other hand, they criticize the lack of transparency on the funding because there was no specific, identified budget. This situation prevents any evaluation process on what constitutes effective spending to improve the quality of life of people with Alzheimer's disease and their families. During this process the year 2007 is designated as 'The Year for Alzheimer' at a national level.

Learning from the past

A national expert committee was set up in August 2007 to evaluate the situation in France and to propose recommendations for the future. This demonstrated the Government's commitment to tackling the problem of dementia. Led by Professor Joël Ménard, a wide consultation was undertaken, including family carers; advocacy, independent and third sector provider organizations; professional bodies; and academic and research experts. Working groups, interviews and audits were carried out. This mechanism encouraged real national debate and promoted opportunities to learn from the past.

Seven years of Alzheimer plans have mainly contributed to raise awareness of dementia in France, and have succeeded in implementing a network of memory clinics throughout the country. One of the characteristics of the second plan was the significant development of day care centres, although not yet enough to meet current needs. Concern for carers' health remained a key theme, as well as the need to increase staff knowledge and skills. Research remained on the agenda for all three plans.

The consultation process of Ménard's Committee identified a continued lack of efficient solutions in terms of diagnosis, treatment, information and support for family caregivers, respite provisions, continuity of care at home, and adapted settings within nursing homes. The issues of information and rights following diagnosis disclosure and throughout the entire journey with dementia have remained a major concern since 2001. The weakness of research, specifically on psychosocial issues, was also identified. The complexity of the health and social care system in France was underlined. Concerning funding, it is now known that there was confusion between the budget supposedly dedicated to the Alzheimer plan and that allocated to other national priorities for older people. After the dramatic events in 2003 when 15,000 older people died in France as a result of exceptional heat during several weeks of summer, an 'Aging and Solidarity' national plan was adopted in November 2003 with a budget of 9.38 million euros dedicated mainly to:

- facilitating home care, increasing the number of home nursing care services, domiciliary care services, respite care facilities and day care centres

- improving medical and nursing care in residential care homes with an increased number (20%) of nurses and auxiliary nurses. In addition 200 new nursing homes will be created and financed. Improving the quality of existing nursing home buildings is also a priority.

In June 2006 this was followed by a new plan: the Old Age and Solidarity Plan. This new plan was focused again on improving home care, residential care provision and hospital wards for old people, with significant funding provided.

In reality the two general plans that focused on older people created confusion in terms of what is financed, in which budget. The lack of transparency prevented any clear evaluation of results for either set of plans.

In November 2007, Professor Joël Ménard presented his report (Ménard 2007) to the president of the French Republic with recommendations for renewed public policy on dementia. The title of the document that summarised the whole approach centred on the person with dementia and their relatives: 'For the patient and his relatives: investigate, cure and care.'

The third Alzheimer plan

In February 2008 the third Alzheimer plan was launched with a total budget of 1.6 billion euros over the period 2008–2012. The French president, Nicolas Sarkozy, launched the plan, stating that 'to fight this illness is a challenge. It has nothing to do with left- or right-wing politics. All governments over the next 30 years will be confronted by it' (Alzheimer Europe 2008a, p.22). Due to criticisms about the management of the previous plans, there was a significant change in the governance structure. An Interministerial Mission was established to monitor the delivery of the plan. To facilitate links between different ministries, national agencies and all stakeholders involved, and to support their actions, the leadership was given to a small core team led by Florence Lustman. The 'Plan Alzheimer Mission' was tasked with evaluating the implementation and controlling the use of the funding dedicated to the plan. A National Steering Committee was also established to regularly monitor the achievements and barriers in the implementation of different actions. To increase transparency, the website of the plan (www.plan-alzheimer.gouv.fr) gives the results of the delivery action by action, including information on the amount of the budget spent on each action.

The third plan has 11 objectives and 44 measures, organised around three main axes:

- *Axis 1:* Improve quality of life for people with dementia and their caregivers.
- *Axis 2:* Improve knowledge for action.
- *Axis 3:* Change perceptions of the public around a key societal issue.

It is not within the scope of this chapter to examine all 44 measures of the third Alzheimer plan, so key aspects of the work in progress three years after the launch of the plan will be presented. The chapter focuses on actions that have improved and/or brought changes in the field of dementia care. Most of the actions commented on relate to the Fondation Médéric Alzheimer's mission, in which the author has been involved in terms of expertise for the implementation and the preparation of guidelines where relevant.

Some of the results[1]

Improving quality of life for people with dementia and their caregivers

This axis alone covers 20 of the 44 measures in the plan, demonstrating the importance attached to supporting a good quality of life for people with dementia and their families. A few of these measures are detailed below.

MEASURE 1: DEVELOPING AND DIVERSIFYING RESPITE CARE PROVISION

This is one of the crucial issues to offer a better quality of life. The aim is to propose a wide range of respite facilities in each area corresponding to the needs of people with dementia and their carers, and to guarantee easier access to these new services. A further aim is to implement solutions that meet individual needs for periods of respite, which are also an opportunity for evaluation and increased social life for the people involved. The plans for day care centres are considered to be on track, with more than 1,663 centres now open in France at the end of 2010 compared to 963 in January 2008. Some new centres are still in the process of development. Nevertheless it has been necessary to better qualify and structure day care centres in order to make them more visible, more accessible and truly efficient for the clients. Studies of implementation and evaluation of these services will go on till the end of 2011. In addition to the development and improvement of day care centres, seen as a central service for respite, the Alzheimer plan focuses on two further objectives:

1. *Encouraging innovative respite provision:* This might include respite at home with 24-hour cover; overnight care teams; short-break holidays; social and cultural outings, and so on. These ideas come from a national study including working groups and interviews with clients and providers. This ongoing work aims to identify a methodology for implementing such new projects for France, as well as establishing the conditions for their successful achievement. To improve and develop best practice for respite, 18 existing respite projects have been selected to be part of a national evaluation programme.

2. *Experimenting with a 'single point of contact' for respite, called 'support and respite platforms':* This aims to address the needs of both caregiver and the person cared for. A respite 'platform' is intended to offer an

---

1   All the figures mentioned in this chapter come from the Steering Committee document of 24 March 2011, available at www.plan-alzheimer.gouv.fr.

extended range of services including call centre, information, support, day care centre, short-term respite stay, holidays, social activities, and so on. Eleven experimental 'platforms' were created in different regions in 2009. At a local level, the platform delivers a diverse but integrated range of options for respite and support for both people with dementia and their caregivers. Over the period 2009–2011 the platforms have been tested and evaluated. Depending on the results from these evaluations and the possibilities for financing, they might be made permanent and serve as models for creating more similar projects.

These developments in respite care were supported by the conclusions of two studies carried out in 2008: one by Gérontopôle (Villars *et al.* 2009) and one by the Fondation Médéric Alzheimer (Villez *et al.* 2008) following a request from the French Ministry of Social Affairs. The Gérontopôle study underlined the lack of evidence on the benefits of respite and recommended improvements in the evaluation of such interventions. The second study established a typology of different respite options supported by a review of French and international literature. Systematic analysis of 400 scientific articles on respite, published between 1990 and 2008, was combined with analysis of the initiatives supported, known and identified by the Fondation Médéric Alzheimer's team in France and abroad. This review showed that betweeen 2000 and 2008 respite options developed through more refined and more targeted segmentation of proposals according to age, degree of autonomy, home situation and socio-cultural characteristics. These 'second-generation' options are more flexible (forms of access, activities), bring services closer to home and take into account the concerted interests of the carer and the person with dementia. A functional typology describes these new approaches: combining several kinds of assistance to reinforce effectiveness; working on the caring/cared-for relationship; taking into account the issues that concern couples; working through networks; reducing tension through family therapy; offering time for socialization; and promoting interventions based on team mobility for people and their families.

MEASURE 2: CONSOLIDATING RIGHTS AND TRAINING FOR CARERS

This is intended to increase support for family members committed to supporting their relative on a daily basis. The necessity of information, knowledge and basic skills is identified as part of the pair's quality of life. Carers' rights and access to training is also reinforced. Two days' training a year are being offered to each family carer. The programme covers the person with dementia, the carer relationship, care advice, non-verbal communication and stress management. The training began in 2010 with the expertise of

France Alzheimer; nevertheless it remains difficult to reach the families (only 2620 people have taken part). An effort needs to be made to guarantee the achievement of this action by wider dissemination and more training centres.

Measure 4: Identification and labelling throughout the country of single points of contact aiming to facilitate integrated care

This is one of the more high-profile actions carried out by the Alzheimer plan. The points of contact are known as *Maisons pour l'Autonomie et l'Intégration des Malades Alzheimer (MAIA)*. A better integration between home and nursing care, memory clinics and information and support structures is supported in order to enable a personalized care pathway to be provided for each person with dementia. Several projects have been implemented in France over the last 20 years to try to respond to the lack of coordination. Based on the principle of integration, the *MAIA* is an attempt to simplify the organization of available care and support options at the level of a given area. Actors in the health, medical and social sectors are encouraged through this new system to get together and coordinate their activities and share information on the individuals concerned. Since 2009, 15 *MAIA* have been established and are currently being evaluated. In early 2011, 40 new *MAIA* were selected for implementation so that 55 *MAIA* will be available by the end of 2011.

Measure 5: Establishing 'Case managers' throughout the country

This is in order to deal with more problematic situations. Working within a *MAIA*, the case manager acts as go-between, providing a link with the various care professionals at the local level to ensure that people with dementia and their relatives obtain a clear and efficient care plan. This unique correspondent, responsible for the care provided as a whole, is seen as the direct contact for the person with dementia, their family and the family doctor. His or her long-term mission, including any episodes in hospital, covers both the health and social aspects of care, such as evaluating and elaborating an individual care plan, and following up actions taken. There are some feelings of dissatisfaction about the *MAIA* and case managers, due to recent history. Many local projects working in line with public policy for older people were already working quite successfully in terms of coordination in spite of problems of funding. The *MAIA* scheme is more ambitious with the aim of integrated care, but it is not yet clear where it will be possible to substitute a *MAIA* in every area where a coordination project is functioning.

MEASURE 6: REINFORCING SUPPORT AT HOME – ADVOCATING SERVICES BY TRAINED STAFF; AND MEASURE 20: A SPECIFIC CAREER AND SKILLS DEVELOPMENT PLAN FOR ALZHEIMER'S DISEASE

In France around 60 per cent of people with dementia live at home (Rocher and Lavallart 2009). That is why these measures are essential. The creation of training for 'gerontological care assistants' should contribute to the improvement of quality of life for people with dementia. Training adapted to the specific psychological challenges of dementia is delivered in the form of continuing training (Aquino, Lavallart and Mollard 2011). Thirty-nine Pilot Specialised Nursing Care teams (Measure 6), including gerontological assistants, psychomotor therapists and occupational therapists, were in place by the end of 2009. By 1 March 2011 a total of 114 teams were working, which is an encouraging sign of success (even if the goal of 500 teams by the end of 2012 will be difficult to achieve). These newly created services offer both treatment and personal assistance. They complement the existing nursing care at home teams already in place for older people. These specialist teams focus on rehabilitation within the person's own environment over a limited period of a few weeks, introducing a new way of looking at the person's capacities and also encouraging creativity by including the family carers.

MEASURE 16: CREATING SPECIFIC UNITS FOR PATIENTS SUFFERING FROM BEHAVIOURAL PROBLEMS WITHIN NURSING HOMES

This aims to improve residential care for better quality of life for people with Alzheimer's. The objective is to create new units or adapt existing units for people with dementia who experience behavioural problems while living in nursing homes. Research finds that 25 per cent of residents have moderate behavioural problems – measured on an internationally validated scale – and 10 per cent have major problems such as aggressiveness, and so on. To address the needs of these residents, the plan evokes 'units reinforced in terms of staffing, with a high level of supervision, the intervention of professionals specially trained, due to the specific nature of the care required' (Alzheimer Europe 2008b). The architecture and layout must also be adapted.

Two kinds of units are in the plan. First, centres for adapted activities and care (*Pôles d'activités et de soins adaptés: PASA*). These are specially adapted treatment and activity units that will be created to offer residents with behavioural problems social and therapeutic activities during the day in a specially adapted living area. Staff in these units will include 'gerontological assistants' with the new skills profile described above (Alzheimer Europe

2008b). Psychomotor, occupational and speech therapists will also be part of the team. By March 2011, 145 *PASA* had been created, and there are 600 planned in total.

Second, reinforced housing units (*Unités d'hébergement renforcées: UHR*). For people with very considerable behavioural problems, reinforced structures will be developed in the form of small units able to house about a dozen people, providing both accommodation and activities and satisfying all the criteria for a suitable care and activity unit. By March 2011, 32 *UHR* had been created, and there are 100 planned in total.

The project to place dedicated day care units within residential settings is also relevant in discussion of improving residential care. The project enables residents with dementia, while keeping their own room, to receive special attention during the day in a dedicated space. The scheme is intended to preserve a peaceful atmosphere for other residents. This is not a new idea, and several nursing homes already provide such units (Guisset-Martinez and Villez 2010).

There has been some initial evaluation of the *PASA* and *UHR* units. Those that succeeded in getting additional staff for *PASA* (some of the 145 agreed *PASA* did not get an additional budget for staff) report that they regret the dominance of the cognitive behavioural approach rather than a psychosocial approach. The criteria established are based on scales and standards that seem to be applied with rigidity by the inspection body and this doesn't fit with the idea of person-centred care that staff and managers have in mind. A measure of disappointment is perceptible from some managers and staff concerning the actual needs they observe among people with dementia. It is perhaps something that can be improved in the coming years. In addition, improving the quality of existing Special Care Units (SCU) within nursing homes is on the agenda of the plan. So far, some funds have been given to improve buildings and adapt environmental settings, but the result is far below expectations.

MEASURE 17: CREATING SPECIALIZED UNITS WITHIN HEALTH CARE REHABILITATION AND FOLLOW-UP DEPARTMENTS FOR ALZHEIMER'S PATIENTS

These are called *Unités cognitive comportementales: UCC*. The *UCC* is a unit of 10 to 12 beds within either generalist or geriatric rehabilitation departments that should offer specific care for both young and older people with dementia, whether they live at home or in an institution. '*UCCs* aim to stabilize behavioural problems using individual cognitive and behavioural rehabilitation programmes and to provide the care given before the crisis situation arises. This cognitive/behavioural specialization in the treatment given to patients with Alzheimer's and related diseases within authorized rehabilitation structures requires the intervention of specific staff (psychomotor therapist, psychologist, occupational therapist, gerontological assistant and so on) and access to psychiatric sessions' (Alzheimer Europe 2008b). By the end of 2010, 41 *UCC* had been created, with 120 planned in total.

MEASURE 18: ACCOMMODATION FOR YOUNG PATIENTS; AND MEASURE 19: IDENTIFYING A NATIONAL REFERENCE CENTRE FOR YOUNG ALZHEIMER'S PATIENTS

Younger people with dementia are a new and important theme of this third French plan. 'The prevalence of early-onset Alzheimer's disease in France is little known. According to data supplied by the state health insurance provider about 8000 people under 60 have "long-term medical condition" (*ALD*) status for Alzheimer's disease' (Alzheimer Europe 2008b). At later stages of the condition, younger people experiencing a loss of autonomy that makes it impossible to remain at home cannot be admitted to the usual health care facilities. A survey is being done by the Fondation Médéric Alzheimer in cooperation with the *Centre National de Référence pour les Malades Alzheimer Jeunes* (*CNR-MAJ* – the national referral centre for younger people with dementia) to find out more about what kinds of care homes younger people live in. Initial results from only two regions find that five in every 1000 young patients live in care homes. National seminars have been conducted on that topic to hear directly what the people concerned want. It has been very interesting to listen to them and the strong opinions they express. It is important to highlight that such a method of empowering the so-called vulnerable client is not normal practice in France.

Measure 19 is dedicated to the national referral centre created for younger people with Alzheimer's or related disorders (*CNR-MAJ*). The goals of this centre are: providing information and increasing awareness of early-onset Alzheimer's among medical and paramedical professionals and others; improving the aetiological and genetic diagnosis; improving care plans; and promoting research and international partnerships. The Lille University Medical Centre and Lille Nord de France University is the *CNR-MAJ* coordinator (www.centre-alzheimer-jeunes.com).

MEASURE 37: STUDYING DISEASE KNOWLEDGE AND ATTITUDES

This aims to change images and attitudes towards Alzheimer's disease. In France, a study within the framework of the 2008 Alzheimer plan revealed that 27 per cent of the population considered it one of the three most serious diseases, while 31 per cent of those over age 18 said they felt or would feel uncomfortable in the presence of someone with Alzheimer's disease. People questioned about the disease used expressions like 'loss of identity, degradation' (22%) and 'scourge, helplessness' (14%), illustrating fear and stigma among the general population in France. Since 2008, seven surveys have been carried out by the *Institut National de Prévention et d'Education Sanitaire (INPES)*, including the general public, people with dementia and professionals working at home. These studies (Pin le Corre *et al.* 2009) are a good way of understanding what people's understanding is, what wishes they express, and what could be future improvements.

MEASURE 38: CREATING A NATIONAL REFERENCE CENTRE ON ETHICS ABOUT ALZHEIMER'S (EREMA)

Since the first Alzheimer plan, ethics is a key issue. Work began in 2003 with a series of regional Round Tables aiming to facilitate the identification of crucial questions and to establish recommendations to preserve the person's dignity. 'Ethics cannot be reduced to professional standards, to simple observance of rules or prefabricated guidelines. Ethics are a goal, a daily quest, never a state or a definitive answer. This is the very nature of ethical reflection' (Ménard 2007) was a statement of Ménard's Commission Report. The National Reference Centre provides a website (www.espace-ethique-alzheimer.org) in which everyone can find information, including videos of conferences, a list of the latest publications and a monthly national and international press review on ethics, prepared by the Fondation Médéric Alzheimer. *EREMA* also organizes workshops, continuing training, and a first Summer University was held in September 2011 in cooperation with the Regional Ethical Centres of Marseille. *EREMA* offers real support for professional carers trying to translate general ethical principles into good daily practices.

MEASURE 42: MAKING THE FIGHT AGAINST ALZHEIMER'S DISEASE A PRIORITY FOR THE EUROPEAN UNION DURING THE FRENCH PRESIDENCY

This aims to invite member states and the European Commission to share national and local experience in the areas of improving diagnosis, medico-social care, integrating care and services, drug strategies and the quality of life of patients and carers. That is why in October 2008 a European Conference was organized in Paris entitled 'The Fight against Alzheimer's Disease and Related Disorders'. In November 2010 a second European Conference, 'Improving the Quality of Life of People with Dementia: A Challenge for European Society', was organized by the Belgian Presidency of the European

Union. It was based on the excellent report of the King Baudouin Foundation (2010). Once again, this event and all the other actions happening at a European level show that a dynamic process has begun.

Table 6.1 Third French Alzheimer Plan actual expenditures 2008–2010 (million €)

Measure	2008	2009	2010	Planned budget 2008–2012
1 (new) respite action	8,60	15,40	13,90	169,50
2 training carers	-	0,10	0,50	12,50
4 MAIA	-	3,864	4,053	27,90
6 nursing home care team	-	1,50	10,20	169
16 PASA	-	-	3,70	228
16 UHR	-	-	6,90	210
16 SCU buildings improvement	-	0	15,40	180
17 UCC	2,40	7,00	8,20	90
19 national reference centre for young Alzheimer's patients	-	0,11	0,357	3
20 gerontological assistant	-	-	0,506	0
37 disease knowledge and attitudes	0,10	-	-	0,10
38 national reference centre on ethics about Alzheimer's	-	0,40	0,10	2
40 ethics workshops	-	0,03	-	0,20

Source: Steering committee 2011 March 24th

Discussion

More than three years after the third Alzheimer plan was launched, several key changes can be observed. People living with dementia are less often seen as patients and more often as people. In some countries, people with dementia speak publicly at conferences and on television programmes. These individuals include Christine Bryden, Peter Ashley, James McKillop and Richard Taylor.

All have done a lot around the world to let us know what it means to live with dementia. In France so far, this is a very new and quite exceptional idea. Nevertheless, the situation is starting to change, mostly thanks to the younger people with dementia. Supported by the focus the plan put on younger people with dementia, they now act to make their voice heard.

Unfortunately, for the majority of people with dementia, often those who are older, it is still a 'silent world' around them. The images of loss and the fears attached to Alzheimer's disease provoke stigma within the family, among the general public and even among professionals. A recent study entitled 'The person's rights in the process of transfer to a care home' (Fondation Médéric Alzheimer 2009) shows that involving people with Alzheimer's disease in the decisions that concern them demands that care providers be attentive to every expression, including non-verbal, in order to perceive any communication by the individual. In daily practice to date it appears to be difficult to respect a person's rights and choices when there is cognitive impairment and problems of communication.

The three Alzheimer plans published in the past ten years have produced some changes and improvements. One of them is a significant evolution in the respite care approach. It was initially perceived as the solution to support family carers coping with a burden. Nowadays, respite practices are diversified, and include activities dedicated to the person with dementia as well as the carers. Respite programmes propose solutions that benefit both people with dementia and their family carers.

In the last few years, views about life with dementia have slowly changed, showing that a good quality of life can continue if some pre-conditions are fulfilled. Social and psychosocial aspects of dementia and a focus on remaining capacities are a little more taken into account. However, the input made by the cognitive-behavioural approach emphasized in the third plan brings the risk that, again, only deficits will be valued, which will not help to remove the stigma attached to dementia. Similarly for research, which includes four measures within the last plan, the main focus is on medical aspects. Psychosocial research teams are still not well committed and recognized in dementia care in France.

The third plan set up very ambitious objectives and it appears that for several measures the results are lower than expected, especially in relation to the experience of the person with dementia. This is partly due to the fact that perhaps too many actions were proposed within a short period. Another obstacle is that since 2008 the organization of social and health care administration has been in a period of change. Regional Health Agencies (*Agences Régionales de Santé*) have been set up since July 2009, and slowly everybody is learning the new decision-making process and becoming able to identify the new key people at the regional level. Many of the new actions and programmes resulting from the plans, except for day care centres, are still being evaluated, although these include initiatives which have been functioning for many years. This is the case for overnight care teams at home, short respite stays, social programmes and leisure activities for people with dementia and their family carers.

Overall the important effort made by France to continue putting dementia on the public and policy agenda is a success. Improvements have been seen and significant funding has been committed to develop the plans' action, but for some measures a significant delay has been experienced and underspending is evidenced; see Table 6.1. It seems clear that the funds dedicated for the third plan have been used as intended, but it is obvious that 1.6 billion euros will not be spent by the end of 2012. The administrative obstacles and organizational difficulties that need to be overcome in order to achieve all the announced actions have slowed down the implementation process. Another reason is that some local stakeholders may be reluctant to create new programmes (e.g. the respite platforms), as there is no guarantee of continuity of public funding after the experimental phase of the action.

The national plan for older people, *Plan Solidarité Grand Age (PSGA)*, mentioned above, is also ongoing. It shares the aims of improving home care and residential homes for older people. These are obviously areas that will also benefit people with dementia. Therefore some of the money from the *PSGA* has been diverted to cover actions from the Alzheimer plans. Some might argue that focusing on dementia for ten years may have prevented adoption of a wider perspective of care for older and younger, vulnerable people. Lessons from the three Alzheimer plans suggest that integrated plans for a broader range of people, including people with dementia, would be a more productive and beneficial approach. Lessons learnt in providing best practice for dementia care can be shared with professionals and practitioners working with adults with a range of needs.

References

Alzheimer Europe (2008a) 'France pledges Euro 1.6 billion to fight Alzheimer's disease.' *Dementia in Europe 1*, 20–22. Available at www.alzheimer-europe.org/upload/SPTUNFUYGGOM/downloads/1D3D25D87428.pdf

Alzheimer Europe (2008b) 'Dementia in Europe: Third Alzheimer Plan.' Available at www.plan-alzheimer.gouv.fr/IMG/pdf/plan-alzheimer-2008-2012.pdf, pp.20–22.

Alzheimer Grande Cause Nationale (2007) *Programme pour les personnes souffrant de la maladie d'Alzheimer et de maladies apparentées*. Available at www.gouvernement.fr/gouvernement/alzheimer-grande-cause-nationale-2007

Aquino, J., Lavallart, B. and Mollard, J. (2011) *Assistant de soins en gérontologie. Le manuel officiel de la formation*. Paris: Elsevier Masson, Alzheimer and Fondation Médéric Alzheimer.

Fondation Médéric Alzheimer (2009) 'The person's rights in the process of transfer to a care home.' *Lettre de l'Observatoire des Dispositifs*, No. 11 (October). Available at www.fondation-mederic-alzheimer.org

Girard, J. and Canestri, A. (2000) *La Maladie d'Alzheimer.* Paris: Ministère de l'Emploi et de la Solidarité.

Guisset-Martinez, M. and Villez, M. (2010) *Regaining Identity: New Synergies, New Approaches to Alzheimer's.* Guide Repères series. Paris: Fondation Médéric Alzheimer.

King Baudouin Foundation (2010) *Improving the Quality of Life of People with Dementia: A Challenge for European Society.* Report in preparation for a high-level conference on dementia in the framework of the Belgian EU Presidency 2010, commissioned by the Belgian Federal Public Service for Health, Food Chain, Safety and Environment. Brussels: King Baudouin Foundation.

Ménard, J. (2007) *Pour le malade et ses proches: Chercher, soigner et prendre soin. Commission Nationale chargée de l'élaboration de propositions pour un plan national concernant la maladie d'Alzheimer et les maladies apparentées.* Report to the President, 8 November 2007.

Pin le Corre, S., Benchiker, P.S., David, M., Deroche, C., Louassarn, S. and Scodellaro, C. (2009) 'Social representations of Alzheimer's disease: The multiple faces of forgetfulness.' *Gérontologie et société 128– 129,* 75–88.

Reynish, E., Bickel, H., Fratiglioni, L., Kiejna, A., Prince, M., Georges, J. and EuroCoDe Prevalence Group (2009) 'Systematic review and collaborative analysis of the prevalence of dementia in Europe.' *Alzheimer's and Dementia 5,* 4, Supplement 1, 393.

Rocher, P. and Lavallart, B. (2009) 'Le Plan Alzheimer 2008–2012.' *Gérontologie et société 128–129,* 13–31.

Table Ronde de Monsieur le Président de la République (2011) *Dossier de presse: Table Ronde de Monsieur le Président de la République consacrée au bilan du Plan Alzheimer 2008–2012.* Paris: Présidence de la République.

Villars, H., Gardette, V., Sourdet, S., Andrieu, S. and Vellas, B. (2009) *Evaluation des structures de répit pour le patient atteint de maladie d'Alzheimer (et syndrome apparenté) et son aidant principal: revue de la littérature.* Toulouse: Gérontopôle de Toulouse.

Villez, M., Ngatcha-Ribert, L., Kenigsberg, P., Guisset-Martinez, M. and Charras, K. (with Michèle Frémontier of the Fondation Médéric Alzheimer, and with the collaboration of Professors Antoine Hennion and Jean-Luc Novella, members of the Comité d'orientation of Fondation Médéric Alzheimer) (2008) *Analyse et revue de la littérature française et internationale sur l'offre de répit aux aidants de personnes atteintes de la maladie d'Alzheimer ou de maladies apparentées.* (Analysis and review of French and international literature on available respite options for caregivers of people with dementia.) Paris: Fondation Médéric Alzheimer.

Chapter 7

Implementing a Regional Strategy

THE FIFE DEMENTIA STRATEGY

Louise McCabe

Introduction

This chapter presents a case study of the Fife Dementia Strategy, a regional dementia strategy from the east of Scotland. The chapter outlines the development of the strategy, commenting on the context for this development and describing the work of the dementia strategy team who put the strategy together. The latter part of the chapter discusses the implementation of the strategy and provides examples of work being undertaken within Fife that has resulted from, or been influenced by, the strategy and the work of the dementia strategy team. This chapter is interesting as it demonstrates the impact of policy and planning at a local level and emphasises the need for involvement of a wide range of stakeholders in local policy processes.

Background: Why develop a local strategy?

Historically, people with dementia have not been considered as a priority group within policy in the United Kingdom (UK) and other countries. Cook (2008) reviewed policy in Scotland and England and found that until 2007 there had been little mention of dementia in policy. Prior to this, the *National Service Framework for Older People* (Department of Health [DH] 2001) was one of the few documents that discussed the needs of people with dementia and recommended specialist services for them. More recently, however, it would appear that activity in the field of dementia care and treatment has reached a point where there is a recognised need at governmental levels for specific policy to address the needs of people with dementia and their carers. There also seems to be political will in many countries to address these issues. This increasing awareness and willingness to act are no doubt linked to the predicted dramatic rise in the numbers of people with dementia (Alzheimer's

Disease International 2010) and to changes in our understanding of dementia care and the needs of people with dementia and their carers.

Across the world the numbers of people with dementia are increasing due to the aging of the population and to improved techniques to identify and diagnose dementia earlier than before, as well as to changing lifestyle factors (Alzheimer's Disease International 2010). In parallel to increasing numbers of people with dementia there has been a shift in understanding of how to care for people with dementia. This has been influenced by research in dementia studies, with recognition that dementia is not simply a disease requiring treatment; instead, people with dementia need individualised support encompassing psychological, social and biomedical aspects of the condition. Kitwood's (1997) work on personhood and person-centred care has been particularly influential in the UK in presenting an alternative approach to caring for people with dementia, and more recently the ethos of personalisation has been promoted for people with dementia with a focus on self-directed support (Alzheimer Scotland 2010). Self-directed support means individuals taking more control of the services and support they receive, often through having more control over the budgets allocated for their care.

These different factors have led to a growing recognition of a need to change the ways in which people with dementia and their informal carers are supported, with a stronger focus on home and community and a move away from institutional care. Responses to these changes are evidenced in the growing number of regional and national dementia strategies and plans in countries across Europe and further afield, such as those published in Scotland (Scottish Government 2010) and Norway (Norwegian Ministry of Health and Care Services 2008).

The Fife Dementia Strategy is a regional dementia strategy developed with the aim of improving the treatment, support and care provided for people with dementia living in the region of Fife in Scotland. Fife is a large local authority area in the east of Scotland with a population of 363,460 that encompasses rural and small urban areas. In line with the rest of the UK, the number of people living with dementia in Fife is set to increase dramatically over the next 20 years. Currently in Fife there are an estimated 5700 people with dementia. Approximately 63.5 per cent of these people live in their own home in the community, while the remaining 36.5 per cent live in long-term care (Knapp *et al.* 2007). Based on demographic predictions, by 2030 the number of people with dementia in Fife will nearly double to an estimated 11,000 people (Reynish *et al.* 2009).

The strategy was developed in response to a recognised need for services to adapt to the increasing number of people with dementia in Fife and the shifting culture of care centred on the home and community. In parallel with this was a need to find cost efficiencies to ensure that increasing numbers of people with dementia could be cared for within existing budgets. The current cost of health, social care and accommodation for people in Fife living with dementia is an estimated £88.6 million per year; by 2030 this will have increased to over £178.7 million per year at today's prices. Informal carers provide much of the care that people with dementia receive, and it has been estimated that the care and support that carers in Fife provide is worth over £49.8 million per year (Fife Council, NHS Fife and Dementia Services Development Centre 2009). Better planning of services and support for people with dementia could help address some of these financial challenges.

The Fife Dementia Strategy was developed at a time of intense political activity in the field of dementia treatment and care. It was developed at the same time as the English national strategy, *Living Well with Dementia* (DH 2009), and both were published in 2009. During this period there were two major national projects taking place in Scotland relating to dementia care. A HEAT (Health improvement, Efficiency, Access and Treatment) target was set, to increase dementia diagnosis by 33 per cent by March 2011 and to improve early diagnosis and management for people with dementia (Scottish Government 2008). To support this target, funding was provided through a scheme called the Mental Health Collaborative to support a range of projects including those for people with dementia. In Fife those projects included work to audit the information given to people following a dementia diagnosis, and a project to increase rates of diagnosis through streamlining referral systems and working with general practitioners (GPs) to improve referral rates. In addition the Integrated Care Pathways (ICP) project was tasked with developing ICPs for a range of conditions, one being dementia. The importance of this project has been highlighted by the Scottish Government's pledge to accelerate this process for dementia as part of the national dementia strategy (Scottish Government 2011). The Fife Dementia Strategy slightly preceded the national strategy in Scotland that was launched in June 2010 (Scottish Government 2010). All three strategies share similar aims and objectives: to improve public awareness and reduce stigma; to improve early diagnosis and support for people with dementia; and to improve the quality of care and support for people with dementia.

Developing the Fife Dementia Strategy

A formal project was set up to develop the Fife strategy. This was a collaborative project between Fife Social Work Services, NHS Fife and the Dementia Services Development Centre, University of Stirling. The project was funded through the Knowledge Transfer Partnership (KTP) scheme (www.ktponline.

org.uk) and ran from January 2008 to December 2009. Development of the strategy was driven by service managers within health and social work looking to improve dementia care across Fife and to plan for future increases in numbers of people with dementia. It is also likely that they were influenced by growing recognition in national governments across the UK of the need for improved dementia care. They lobbied support from policy makers in the region and sought out funding through the KTP scheme to take their plan forward. The funding for this project provided a full-time post, the knowledge transfer associate, and input from academics at the University of Stirling. Staff members from Fife Social Work Services and NHS Fife were also assigned to coordinate the project.

The first year of the project involved information gathering from local sources and published literature as well as policy from the UK and further afield to identify good practice in dementia care and treatment. There was also extensive consultation with different stakeholders within Fife as to what was needed to improve services and support for people with dementia and their carers. These stakeholders included professionals and practitioners as well as people with dementia, their carers and other service users. Most of this work was done by the knowledge transfer associate through individual meetings and attendance at existing meetings across Fife. In addition two stakeholders' events were held in the first year of the project, bringing together around 100 practitioners and professionals at each event. These events were utilised to disseminate information about the strategy development and to gather views and opinions from those attending.

It was decided during the first year that a group of key stakeholders from across Fife should be brought together to form a working group to guide the development of the strategy; this group was named the Dementia Strategy Working Group (DSWG). The DSWG was a multidisciplinary and multiagency group with 22 members. Members utilised their expertise combined with research and good practice evidence to develop a series of recommendations that informed the specific development of the strategy. The DSWG met seven times, and an additional 17 local experts attended when relevant over the course of the meetings, and corresponded multiple times over email. The group discussed a series of topics relating to dementia care and support, using research evidence to work out ways to improve services on the ground. The topics under discussion covered the range of support and services currently available to people with dementia in Fife and followed the journey of a person with dementia from public awareness and diagnosis through to end-of-life care. The development of the Fife Dementia Strategy also benefited from the contributions of service providers and users from across Fife, particularly during the consultation process described below.

In July 2009, during the second year of the project, a draft strategy and consultation document were developed and a wide-ranging consultation process took place to collect the views of as broad a range of stakeholders as possible. The draft strategy was split into sections relating to different types of care and support and roughly followed the expected journey of someone with dementia from diagnosis, through services at home and institutional care to end-of-life care. Each section included a summary of current provision in Fife; a series of outcomes and recommendations to improve services in that specific area for people with dementia; and an action plan to achieve these outcomes. The consultation process took place over a six-week period.

A range of techniques was adopted to encourage participation in this process. A consultation document was prepared, presenting the draft strategy and asking people to respond. The consultation document was made available in different forms: a full version and an abridged version; large type face was available on request or the strategy could be sent electronically. The document could be accessed through the internet and local networks for social work, health and housing staff. In addition hard copies were posted to all independent sector care home providers. The local Alzheimer Scotland office was also closely involved. The consultation was advertised by placing posters in public places including post offices and GP surgeries. By the time of the consultation many stakeholders within health and social work were aware of the strategy and helped disseminate the consultation document. Stakeholders in Fife were asked to comment on the proposed recommendations, actions and outcomes, and to help identify how each might be achieved. A detailed series of questions was provided to encourage focused responses.

At this time the project team was aware that just a few people with dementia had been consulted directly during the development of the strategy and it seemed unlikely that many would respond to the written and internet calls for responses. It was, however, felt to be essential that people with dementia were included. To address this gap a series of group interviews were planned with people with dementia, other service users and carers. Following ethical approval from the Local Research Ethics Committee, a series of eight group interviews took place during the consultation, involving 56 service users, 14 of whom were identified by staff as people with dementia, five family carers and nine staff members. The aim of these events was to enable people with dementia and other people using the same services to contribute their views on current services and on the strategy. The group interviews were held in settings where people with dementia and other older service users would normally attend, such as day centres, care homes and community centres. At each location, group interview participants were drawn from that setting and invitations were also sent to family carers living close by. Carers attended four of the focus groups. The groups ranged in size from 7 to 11 participants. Each of the groups had a different mix of people with dementia, older service users, carers and care staff.

Two or three topics were chosen from a list of services and support currently provided for people with dementia in Fife. Topics were chosen according to the expected experiences of participants in each group. Often, however, groups covered a broader range of topics according to the interests of participants. Two researchers facilitated each group to support participation by everyone present. Participants appeared to enjoy the discussion and most took part. Care staff, where involved, often provided support and encouragement for people to participate, although at times they could talk over the service users. Some of the people with dementia we met limited their participation to nods in agreement to others, while others were active contributors to the discussions.

In total, during the whole consultation process, 97 written and verbal responses were received from a broad range of stakeholders including: GPs, carers, social workers, nurses, care home workers, consultants from geriatrics and old age psychiatry, people with dementia and other people using the same services.

The draft strategy and consultation document were generally very well received by public and professionals across Fife. The recommendations and actions for improving dementia services were reported as largely the right ones, and the layout of the strategy was well regarded. However, there was a series of suggestions made by people on how the strategy could be improved, and significant changes were made to the strategy following the consultation process. Examples of the key areas raised by respondents to the consultation exercise were:

- the need for awareness campaigns to promote healthy lifestyles

- the need for a more coordinated and comprehensive approach to training

- improvement necessary in current assessment and diagnosis processes

- a stronger focus needed on early and ongoing health care; the importance of information and advocacy services

- a need for improved transport.

(Ellis 2009)

These issues, among others, were incorporated into the final version of the strategy. This was completed in late 2009 and presented to the elected members of the local council for approval.

The Fife Dementia Strategy

The Fife Dementia Strategy was approved in November 2009 by the local authority Health and Social Care Partnership. The strategy is outcome focused, aimed at improving the quality of care available for people with potential or diagnosed dementia, and has been written for Fife with full consideration given to the local context. The strategy is divided into two broad areas:

1. Improving awareness, knowledge and understanding of dementia in the general public and among professionals throughout Fife.

2. Improving the care and services available for people affected by dementia in Fife.

The full-length strategy included a series of chapters focusing on a type of service or support for people with dementia. Each chapter included some background information and a series of aims and recommendations for the future. The strategy also included a very detailed action plan that set out how each aim and recommendation could be achieved and an estimated timescale for this. The strategy also provided a set of ten-year outcomes for the strategy.[1]

The strategy has 19 aims and 41 recommendations and actions that should lead to nine intended outcomes at the end of the strategy's ten-year plan.

These nine intended outcomes are:

1. Increased collaborative working across all sectors and services who work with people affected by dementia.

2. Increased use of community groups and networks by people with dementia and their carers.

3. Improved access to services.

4. Increased flexibility of services.

5. Increased services which are responsive to individual need.

6. Improved continuity in care.

7. Increased staff knowledge and skill surrounding dementia in all generalist and specialist staff.

8. Increased awareness of dementia.

9. Increased opportunities for carers and people with dementia to be involved in service development and provision with support from advocacy services.

---

1   The full strategy can be accessed at http://socialwork.fife.gov.uk/fds/mod/resource/view.php?id=66.

In addition, the strategy stated that, within ten years, services for people with dementia in Fife would be:

- responsive to the needs of people with dementia and their carers

- guided and developed through the use of individual budgets and self-directed support

- integrated into the community

- operated through joint efforts across health, social care and housing providers

- non-exclusive and based on diagnosis and need

- communicating effectively across and within services, as well as between service users and providers.

(Fife Council, NHS Fife and Dementia
Services Development Centre 2009)

These aims and intended outcomes for the strategy reflect current thinking in dementia care in the UK. They are focused on individuals with dementia, aiming to offer them an individualised service that supports them in making choices about their own care and support and enables them to remain living at home. Long-term aims are to provide more personal options for care within a framework of self-directed support.

Implementation of the strategy

As a regional policy it was important that the strategy fit closely to current delivery of support and services for people with dementia and, to achieve this, detailed action plans were included for each aspect of dementia care covered by the strategy, and these were linked with current service delivery. This is illustrated by some of the early aims of the strategy. These included improved use of assistive technology for people with dementia and review of the carers' strategy to ensure that carers of people with dementia receive the support they need. Assistive technology was already an area that Fife Social Work Services had invested in; therefore, it was a relatively simple step to ensure that people with dementia were seen as a key client group for this service. Fife currently uses assistive technology in innovative ways with people with dementia — for example, a safe walking project using Global Positioning Satellite (GPS) tracking devices. A regional carers' strategy was already in development, and again it was possible to use the dementia strategy to ensure inclusion of carers of people with dementia in the regional carers' strategy.

The first crucial step in implementation was the identification of 'dementia leads' from social work and health within Fife. This was important in ensuring the strategy implementation went forward, and the leads also keep the local council Health and Social Work Partnership up to date with the strategy implementation. The National Audit Office (2010) emphasises the need for empowered leadership to implement the National Dementia Strategy in England, but little evidence was found of this following the initial evaluation of the strategy. Only 21 per cent of psychiatrists reported that a senior clinician had taken a lead in 2009, and very few frontline health and social care staff could identify leaders. This was the first step taken in Fife and one that has ensured that the dementia strategy remains a live document with real commitment from those in positions of responsibility. In addition, the DSWG continued to meet for a year following approval of the strategy and provided updates to the dementia leads on dementia projects in their specific organisations and services. This was coordinated by the academic partner from the original strategy development project.

What is happening now?

The sections below provide short case studies of some of the work currently taking place in Fife that supports people with dementia and their carers. This is just a sample of the various projects currently taking place. The description of the Fife Dementia Showcase gives some idea of the breadth of involvement in Fife with services and support for people with dementia. These projects may not have developed as a direct result of the Fife Dementia Strategy but they have been affected by the focus on dementia across Fife. The work of the strategy development team and the various events associated with this work, including the meetings of the DSWG, two stakeholder events and a launch event in March 2011, have created a buzz in Fife around 'dementia'. Professionals and practitioners working with people with dementia in Fife were given recognition and support to continue and develop their work. The strategy provided evidence for the need to improve and expand services for people with dementia, and ideas for more innovative approaches to care.

Fife Dementia Learning Forum

The Fife Dementia Learning Forum provides education and an opportunity to network for professionals and practitioners across Fife; it is interdisciplinary and invites people from all sectors, as well as family carers of people with dementia and people with dementia themselves. The forum has been running for four years and has managed to secure funding from a range of sources to keep the forum running. Meetings are held six times a year and take place at lunchtimes to facilitate attendance. Meetings start with a presentation from a keynote speaker on a topic chosen by forum members, followed by networking over lunch, then small conversational learning groups to discuss the keynote speaker, share experiences and consolidate learning. The forum continues to grow in popularity and now attracts more members from private and voluntary sectors than previously (Anderson 2011). It is no coincidence that the numbers of people attending have increased during development and following publication of the strategy document. Recent topics for discussion include horticulture, living with risk, acute hospital care, music therapy and doll therapy. Participants report very positively on the forum with comments such as 'very motivational speaker, will implement ideas in my workplace' (Anderson 2011, p.4). The forum is successful in promoting best practice in dementia care and presenting new ideas in an accessible and relevant manner.

Reablement

Across Scotland the concept of reablement is being introduced into home care services for adults. The definition of 'reablement' adopted by the Department of Health's Care Services Efficiency Delivery (CSED) Programme is: 'Services for people with poor physical or mental health to help them accommodate their illness by learning or re-learning the skills necessary for daily living' (Newbronner and Chamberlain 2008). The focus of reablement services is the rehabilitation and re-skilling of individuals to increase their independence and reduce the need for high levels of ongoing care. Home care reablement services are well established in England but don't usually include people with dementia, due to the assumption that people with dementia would not benefit from this type of service. In Scotland, reablement is increasingly being introduced as a part of home care for adults, often with the inclusion of people with dementia. Different approaches are taken, with some areas introducing reablement teams that work alongside other home care teams. In Fife, the decision has been taken to completely restructure home care services, making reablement an integrated feature, and to include people with dementia as service users. All new referrals for home care will go to the reablement team, who offer multidisciplinary assessment and intervention with the aim of increasing skills and independence. This initial phase lasts six weeks and, following this, individuals receive ongoing care from the home care service. The reablement process should eliminate or reduce the level of ongoing care. Over time all home care service users will be offered this six-week reablement service and all home care staff will be trained in reablement techniques. This will mean that even the long-term, ongoing care has a reablement focus and that individuals will continue to be supported to be more independent and develop skills. The lead for the reablement project is also the social work lead for the Fife Dementia Strategy, and as such the reablement project shares and takes forward many of the key objectives of the dementia strategy.

The Fife Dementia Showcase

In June 2011 the Fife Dementia Showcase titled 'Innovative Dementia Practices in Fife' was held. This was a collaborative event set up by NHS Fife and Fife Council with the aim to showcase ongoing work in Fife that supports people with dementia and their carers, in line with the dementia strategy. The showcase included 22 presentations from projects across Fife. Invited speakers talked about using technology to support dementia care, presented an innovative project to support safe walking through the use of GPS devices, and summarised the work of the Mental Health Collaborative for people with dementia, discussed above. The 20 parallel sessions were presented by a broad range of professionals and practitioners from health, social work, housing, advocacy services and care homes, and included people from private, voluntary and statutory services. Topics included cognitive stimulation therapy, life story work, doll therapy, independent advocacy, dementia and vision loss, the role of liaison nurses, palliative care, environmental design, housing support, younger adults with dementia, and telecare. The event was attended by over 100 people from across Fife, including carers and people with dementia as well as health and social care staff. The range and depth of the presentations demonstrated a huge commitment within Fife to promote better care for people with dementia. They also demonstrate what can be done within current financial restrictions, showing how individuals and groups can find ways of working that improve the lives of people with dementia without additional cost. The Fife Dementia Strategy has supported and guided professionals and practitioners in the field and encouraged them to stand up and speak about the often innovative work they are undertaking.

Conclusion

The projects outlined above are just some that demonstrate the depth and breadth of commitment to improving dementia care in Fife. The Fife Dementia Showcase is a clear indication of the amount and diversity of work taking place in Fife. It is clear that these projects and services contribute to meeting the aims and objectives of the strategy, but what is less clear is whether their development was driven by the strategy. There were groups and individuals within social work and health services in Fife who were committed to improving care for people with dementia long before the strategy project was undertaken. There were others just beginning projects that fell into step with the strategy development. The very fact that a drive existed among groups and individuals in Fife to develop a project, secure funding and produce the strategy demonstrates this existing commitment. These individuals were already providing innovative approaches to care and support for people with dementia. The strategy gave further support for their work and approval for the direction of travel from the elected council members. In addition the strategy development project got everyone in Fife talking about dementia; 'dementia' became a buzzword, with enthusiasm and support for developments evident across Fife. Links were also made between sectors and across disciplines through the DSWG and the various events linked to the strategy development. People were able to talk directly to colleagues without the formal referral and communication channels and therefore address issues and problems commonly faced.

Despite the best intentions of health and social care professionals in Fife there are sometimes decisions made that are necessary to meet financial targets, even if they appear to be detrimental to the lives of service users such as people with dementia and in addition go against key aims within the dementia strategy. One such example is the decision taken by the elected members of the local council in Fife to close all ten council-run care homes and replace these with independent sector care homes. The local council care homes that will close have received some of the highest ratings from the Care Commission, the national regulatory body, in the past few years and this decision has come as a blow to the many staff working in the homes, the residents themselves and their families and friends. Hopefully the high level of dementia awareness across Fife and the skills of the staff working within these homes will ensure that these closures and the inevitable transfers for residents are undertaken in such a manner as to minimise negative outcomes for people with dementia and their carers. These changes reflect the shifting nature of policy and highlight the need for clear principles for dementia care to be embedded in the everyday practice of professionals and practitioners working with people with dementia.

This chapter demonstrates the value of local policy development that engages with a broad range of stakeholders and that listens to the views of service users and their carers. The way in which dementia care was prioritised through the work of the strategy group and the development of the strategy has clearly impacted on dementia care across Fife. Individuals and groups have taken responsibility for adapting existing services and developing new approaches to care and treatment to create better local services for people with dementia. The strategy work raised the profile of these individuals and groups and demonstrated the value of their work. It is the engagement and enthusiasm of these practitioners and professionals from health and social work in Fife that will continue to improve the experiences of people with dementia and their carers, rather than the detail of the strategy document. However, the value of the strategy development process should not be underestimated.

References

Alzheimer Scotland (2010) *Let's Get Personal – Personalisation and Dementia.* Edinburgh: Alzheimer Scotland.

Alzheimer's Disease International (2010) *World Alzheimer's Report.* London: Alzheimer's Disease International.

Anderson, S. (2011) *Fife Dementia Learning Forum: Evaluation Report 2010–2011.* Fife: NHS Fife and Fife Council.

Cook, A. (2008) *Dementia and Well Being (Policy and Practice in Health and Social Care Series).* Edinburgh: Dunedin Academic Press.

Department of Health (2001) *National Service Framework for Older People.* London: Department of Health.

Department of Health (2009) *Living Well with Dementia: The National Dementia Strategy.* London: Department of Health.

Ellis, B. (2009) *The Fife Dementia Strategy 2010–2020: Public Consultation Response and Analysis.* Fife: Fife Council.

Fife Council, NHS Fife and Dementia Services Development Centre (2009) *The Fife Dementia Strategy 2010–2020.* Fife: Fife Council. Available at http://socialwork.fife.gov.uk/fds/mod/resource/view.php?id=66 [accessed June 2011].

Kitwood, T. (1997) *Dementia Reconsidered.* Buckingham: Open University Press.

Knapp, M., Prince, M., Albanese, E., Banerjee, S. *et al.* (2007) *Dementia UK.* London: The Alzheimer's Society.

National Audit Office (2010) *Improving Dementia Services in England – An Interim Report.* London: National Audit Office.

Newbronner, R. and Chamberlain, L. (2008) 'Improving independence – can homecare re-ablement make a difference in the long term?' *Community Care,* 19 June. Available at www.communitycare.co.uk/Articles/19/06/2008/108581/Improving-Independence-Can-Homecare-Reablement-Make-a-Difference-in-the-Long.htm [accessed November 2011].

Norwegian Ministry of Health and Care Services (2008) *Dementia Plan 2015.* Oslo: Norwegian Ministry of Health and Care Services.

Reynish, E., Bickel, H., Fratiglioni, L., Kiejna, A., Prince, M., Georges, J. and EuroCoDe Prevalence Group (2009) 'Systematic review and collaborative analysis of the prevalence of dementia in Europe.' *Alzheimer's and Dementia 5,* 4, Supplement 1, 393.

Scottish Government (2008) *HEAT Targets.* Available at www.scotland.gov.uk/Topics/Health/health/mental-health/servicespolicy/DFMH/antidepressantprescribing [accessed June 2011].

Scottish Government (2010) *Scotland's National Dementia Strategy.* Edinburgh: Scottish Government, Available at www.scotland.gov.uk/Publications/2010/09/10151751/0 [accessed June 2011].

Scottish Government (2011) *Scotland's National Dementia Strategy: One Year On Report.* Edinburgh: Scottish Government. Available at www.scotland.gov.uk/Publications/2011/06/01142419/14 [accessed June 2011].

Chapter 8

Challenges of Developing a Dementia Strategy

The Case of Malta

Charles Scerri

Introduction

One of the most important challenges facing Maltese society is the increasing size of the elderly population. As a result, neurodegenerative diseases normally associated with old age, such as many forms of dementia, are expected to rise proportionately. This will bring about a significant demand not only on the health care services but also on society as a whole, as most dementia care in Malta is provided by close relatives living in the community. It is therefore clear that the devastating impact of dementia cannot be ignored, and doing nothing is not an option. Malta needs to invest in high-quality care that would incorporate the various aspects of dementia care, from training health care professionals to building nursing and residential homes specifically designed for individuals with dementia. It is a long-term strategy based on skills, knowledge and hard work involving both professionals and the community.

The recommendations presented in this chapter were the result of wide consultations held with stakeholders coming from various sectors of the Maltese community as well as the Maltese public in general. It is augured that these recommendations will act as a framework on which a national dementia strategy will be implemented in Malta.

Geography, demography and health care structure

The Maltese archipelago consists of three main islands: Malta, Gozo and Comino. It is located in the centre of the Mediterranean Sea with Sicily 93 km to the north and northern Africa 288 km to the south. Its total land area is 315 km², making it the smallest country in the European Union. According to the National Statistics Office, the total population of Malta in 2009 was estimated at 412,970, of which just over half were females.

Malta scores high on the Human Development Index with a current life expectancy of 77.7 years for males and 81.4 years for females. The infant mortality rate is 5.96/1000 live births. The birth rate has been steadily declining and is currently one of the lowest in the Mediterranean countries. The percentage of population aged 65 years and above currently stands at 15 per cent of the general population.

Circulatory diseases are the leading cause of death, accounting for 46 per cent of all deaths and 8 per cent of all hospital admissions. Diabetes is highly prevalent in Malta, a pattern shared with other Mediterranean countries. Within the 25–64 age group, 34 per cent of Maltese women and 22 per cent of Maltese men are obese. At age five, 13 per cent of boys and 11 per cent of girls are obese; at age ten, these figures are 19 per cent and 24 per cent respectively.

Health care in Malta is provided through two systems: statutory and private. Health care in the public sector is highly centralised and regulated. The government delivers primary health care through eight health centres that offer a full range of preventive, curative and rehabilitative services. In secondary and tertiary care, specialised ambulatory care is provided in public outpatient clinics and health centres. The Ministry of Health finances, regulates and acts as service provider for public hospitals. A number of private hospitals are also available. The health sector is one of Malta's largest employers, employing 7 per cent of the total workforce. There are 260 doctors, 550 nurses and 200 pharmacists per 100,000 population.

In recent years, medicines and medical devices have been the fastest-growing component of public health care expenditure in Malta. This is mostly due to ever-increasing medical care needs and the advent of new generations of drugs and products. The government supplies medicines listed in the hospital drug formulary free of charge to all in-patients in public hospitals. Other individuals entitled to free medication include pink and yellow card holders: pink card holders (also referred to as Schedule II patients) benefit under the Medical Aids Grant of the Malta Social Security Act and entitlement is based on the total household income; yellow card holders (also referred to as Schedule V patients) are individuals with a specific chronic condition listed in the Fifth Schedule of the Social Security Act. Unfortunately dementia is not one of the conditions included in this list, and therefore anti-dementia medications are not available free of charge under this system.

Dementia care and support in Malta

A recent study on the prevalence of dementia in Malta showed that there is a clear shift towards a progressively aging population where the percentage of individuals aged 65 years and over will double, reaching 28 per cent by the year 2050 (Abela *et al.* 2007). In 2005, for every individual aged 65 years and over, there were 5.2 people in the working-age population bracket. However, by 2050 this ratio will decline to 1:2.2 (Figure 8.1). This decrease in the workforce will increase further financial pressures on social and health care services that currently are heavily subsidised by the central government.

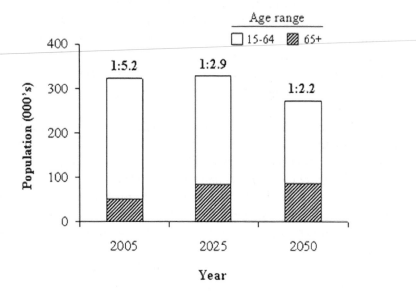

Figure 8.1 Distribution of the total Maltese population according to age brackets for the years 2005, 2025 and 2050[1]

Source: Abela *et al.* 2007

With respect to the prevalence rates of dementia, the estimated total number of dementia cases in 2005 was 4072, an increase of almost 14 per cent from the estimated figure for 2001. The number of individuals with dementia in Malta will significantly increase in 2025 to an estimated total of 6345 and will reach 2 per cent of the general population by 2050 (Table 8.1).

---

1   Numbers in bold atop of the bars denote the old-age dependency ratios. By the year 2050, there will be 2.2 individuals in the working-age bracket for every individual above the age of 65 years.

Table 8.1 Projected number of total dementia cases
in the Maltese islands according to age groups
for the years ranging from 2010 to 2050

Year	Age groups					Total cases	% of total population
	30–59	60–64	65–69	70–74	75+		
2010	203	293	316	629	2947	4388	1.12
2015	204	268	444	749	3227	4892	1.25
2020	201	285	404	1035	3660	5585	1.44
2025	201	253	422	931	4538	6345	1.66
2035	190	257	332	881	5161	6821	1.91
2050	150	268	414	970	4567	6369	2.00

Source: Abela *et al.* 2007

A number of services are available from the Department of Social Services irrespective of whether an individual has dementia or not. These include an age pension to individuals who have attained the retirement age of 61 years; a carer pension (available to individuals who are either single or widowed and are the full-time sole carer of a sick relative who is bedridden or confined to a wheelchair in the same household); a disability pension (available to individuals with a severe disability); and an invalidity pension (for individuals certified as incapable of suitable employment due to serious disease or bodily or mental impairment). Other services intended for the elderly are provided by the Department for the Elderly and Community Care (within the Ministry of Health) and include the provision of day centres with the purpose of preventing social isolation; home help offering non-nursing personal help and light domestic work for older adults and individuals with special needs; telecare; incontinence service; *kartanzjan* (a special card issued to individuals on reaching the age of 60, entitling the holder to obtain rebates and concessions on a number of services such as local transport); meals-on-wheels (to support elderly individuals who are unable to prepare a meal); and a handyman service which offers household repairs. The services offered by both governmental departments are widely available, can be accessed online (www.gov.mt), and are very popular with the elderly, both those living in the community and those in state-run residential care. In terms of care for the elderly and the disabled in general, Malta spent €46 million in 2009 (4% of the total social protection budget), excluding pensions, hospital facilities and other various subsidies (National Statistics Office 2010). No figures for individuals with dementia or their carers availing themselves of such services are currently available.

The Department for the Elderly and Community Care also runs the largest state residential home for elderly people in Malta (St Vincent de Paul's Residence) which accommodates over 1100 residents in approximately 24 hospital-style wards. Due to the increasing needs of individuals with dementia, the residence also houses two dementia wards that are specifically designed for these individuals and manned by staff trained in person-centred dementia care. An activity centre specialised for individuals with dementia and their carers is also located within the premises. This service was launched in 2007 and provides an opportunity for participation and social interaction for residents with dementia, as well as those in the community. Specialised geriatric medical care and rehabilitation services are provided at Karen Grech Hospital and run by a group of interdisciplinary health care professionals. Other services offered by this hospital include the Memory Clinic and respite care, available in special circumstances like hospital admission of the main carer.

Besides government-run homes for the elderly, homes run by the Roman Catholic Church and privately run homes are also available at a cost. With few exceptions, none are designed to cater for the needs of individuals with dementia.

Support within the community comes mostly from the Malta Dementia Society. This non-governmental, non-profit organisation was established in September 2004 on the occasion of World Alzheimer's Day and is run solely by non-paid volunteers. It is intended to offer support primarily for people with dementia and their carers, families and friends, but also brings together health care professionals and other interested parties wishing to learn more about the various aspects of dementia and its care. The main aim of the society is to provide information and to raise awareness about dementia (Scerri and Abela 2006). The society has frequent discussions with the local authorities about ways of enhancing services for individuals with dementia and has been instrumental in establishing various government-run services intended for people with dementia.

Towards a national dementia plan

In May 2009 the Department for the Elderly and Community Care launched the Malta Dementia Strategy Group. The aim of this working group was to devise a number of recommendations that would enhance dementia services and address local shortfalls in dementia care. Its objective was to 'study, advise and recommend the planning and development of services that provide high-quality care for individuals with dementia in the Maltese islands.' The work was carried out by first analysing in detail the services currently available for individuals with dementia and their carers, followed by a wide consultation process with stakeholders working in the field of dementia, and the public in general. The findings were incorporated in a report that also included a number of recommendations serving as a framework for a national plan on dementia. This report was presented to the health authorities in January 2010.

Analysis of existing services

As expected, field analysis on the services available for individuals with dementia showed considerable lack of support for these patients and for those who care for them. This is coupled with a lack of staff trained in patient-centred dementia care. Services that are provided by the various government departments are not tailored for the needs of these individuals, especially if the patient is still relatively young. Academic training tends to focus on the disease model, with continuing education being minimal. In the community, training of carers is only provided by the Malta Dementia Society through a series of organised talks and seminars. These, however, are too few and far between to meet the demand of an ever-increasing number of individuals seeking information about caring. Help in the community is lacking, and individuals with dementia and their carers feel that they are being left to fend for themselves (Innes, Abela and Scerri 2011). The unavailability of free anti-dementia drugs is also putting significant financial strain on the affected families, and most individuals with dementia cannot afford to purchase such medication. Awareness among the general public and the medical profession is lacking, especially in primary care, where general practitioners fail to recognise the symptoms of dementia early, or rather take a wait-and-see approach to diagnosis (Caruana-Pulpan 2010).

Consultation process

The next phase was the launch of the consulation process with stakeholders and the public. The objective of meeting the stakeholders was to get feedback from professional and non-professional bodies that are involved in one or various aspects of dementia management. A number of meetings were organised by the Dementia Strategy Group with stakeholders coming from various sectors of Maltese society, divided into five contact groups:

1. education (including academic bodies coming from various faculties and centres within the University of Malta)

2. professional bodies (including representatives of medical and allied professions)

3. long-term care service providers (including representatives of staff working in state-run and private residential homes and hospitals)

4. acute and intermediate service providers (including representatives of staff working in acute hospital settings)

5. the community (including members of the Malta Dementia Society, the general public, Catholic Church representatives and local council representatives).

For a wider consultation process, the public was invited to send feedback by means of a specifically designed questionnaire that was available online (www.dementia.gov.mt). The structure of the questionnaire was such that it would remain anonymous and could be completed by various categories of the population that might or might not be directly affected by dementia. It was composed of 25 multiple-choice questions on various aspects of dementia awareness, care and management. The questionnaire was widely published in the local media and individuals with no internet access were invited to request a copy by post. Most of the results that will be discussed in this chapter come from in-depth analysis of the data obtained from this part of the consultation process.

Analysis of response to questionnaires

A total number of 613 completed questionnaires were received and analysed. Respondents (71.6% females, 28.4% males) came from all localities of the Maltese islands and consisted of health care professionals (37.7%), direct carers (23.3%), relatives (non-main carers) (5.1%), individuals with dementia (2.8%) and other members of the public (31.1%). Most respondents (63.3%) were in the age range between 30 and 70 years.

Awareness, education and training

Education on the various aspects of dementia is a major pillar in the design of any strategy aimed at providing quality care. Education is also a major tool in increasing awareness about the condition, at a professional level as well as in the community. Educating the public will help eliminate stigma and so promote early diagnosis and management. Unfortunately, in Malta, there is still the belief that dementia is a direct consequence of aging and this misunderstanding commonly acts as a barrier to seeking medical assistance early on in the disease process. During the initial field analysis, it became evident that knowledge about dementia at an undergraduate level is variable, fragmented and lacks focus on the social issues involved in disease progression. Furthermore, there is a lack of educational methods that prepare students to work in interdisciplinary teams or collaboration settings. On a community level, increase in dementia awareness and education is mostly carried out by the Malta Dementia Society through talks, seminars and media campaigns.

Discussion with stakeholders involved in the education and training of health care professionals at both undergraduate and postgraduate levels concluded that:

1. The old medical model of health in dementia care is too restrictive to respond effectively to the multifaceted and diverse nature of dementia.

2. A common ground between the health and social care professions needs to be agreed upon so that students will be able to manage individuals with dementia within a person-centred model of care. This type of care extends beyond the competence of any one profession.

3. Possible steps towards enhancing the competencies of health and social care students with the skills necessary to provide the best quality of dementia care include access to shared study units; organisation of optional credits and multidisciplinary workshops; involvement of students' associations; and facilitation of access to clinical placements within institutions housing individuals with dementia.

Results from the public questionnaire showed that dementia was not considered to be a taboo subject, and therefore the stigma associated with individuals with dementia and their families was diminishing. This was especially evident among the carers, relatives and health care professionals (Figure 8.2). However, the same categories of respondents indicated that awareness about dementia is still lacking (Figure 8.3).

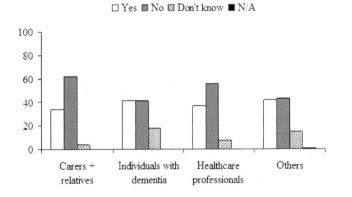

Figure 8.2 Percentage response (vertical axis) from different categories of the Maltese public on whether dementia is still considered to be a taboo subject (N/A = not applicable)

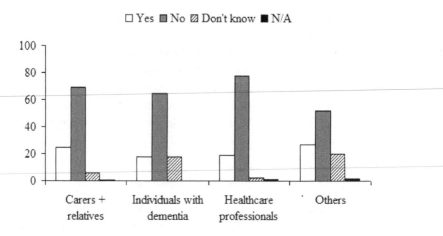

Figure 8.3 Percentage response (vertical axis) from different categories of the public on whether enough awareness on dementia is available in Malta (N/A = not applicable)

Factors that may have hindered individuals from seeking medical advice following the appearance of the first symptoms included the belief that symptoms will pass away (21.6%), presence of social stigma (8.3%) and the belief that such symptoms are to be expected in old age (28.2%).

Only 36 per cent of respondents overall indicated that health care professionals have the necessary skills in dementia care. Notably, the health care profession was the most strongly convinced of the lack of sufficient training in dementia care skills (Figure 8.4).

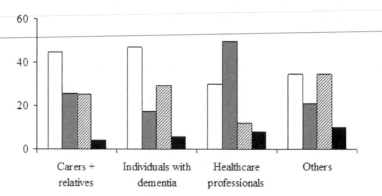

Figure 8.4 Percentage response (vertical axis) from different categories of the Maltese public, indicating whether health care professionals have the necessary skills in dementia care (N/A = not applicable)

In general, although the taboo surrounding dementia is on the decrease, there is still lack of awareness all across the Maltese population. There is also the need to enhance research and training in various areas of dementia care and management by adopting a multidisciplinary approach. Furthering both awareness and education should ultimately lead to a more knowledgeable society that will promote early diagnosis and reduce discrimination.

Box 8.1 Recommendation 1

- *Improve awareness of dementia in the community and in relevant professional and non-professional fields*

This recommendation could be achieved by:

1. Developing targeted information campaigns for the general public.
2. Increasing patient-centred dementia care training for health care professionals.
3. Developing new models of education that emphasise an interprofessional approach in dementia care.
4. Having a 24-hour dementia helpline that acts as a point-of-information reference to the community.

EARLY INTERVENTION

In Malta, the majority of individuals with dementia are not diagnosed early on in the disease process. As a result, diagnosis takes place when the disease has already advanced to a stage that has a significant negative impact on the health and functioning of the affected individual. Understandably, health care professionals need to have the necessary training in identifying the symptoms of dementia and acting accordingly. In a significant number of cases, the first contact for advice is through the family doctor. However, a recent study observed that although the majority of family doctors indicated that they do not have enough training in dementia diagnosis and management, few refer patients to specialist care – with the result that individuals in the early stages of dementia are being deprived of a possible timely diagnosis and early pharmacological intervention (Caruana-Pulpan 2010). Following personal feedback from individuals with dementia, their carers and medical professionals, the Malta Dementia Strategy Group recommends that a state-run central point should exist where proper diagnosis and support are available to the public, especially for those who cannot afford private specialised medical consultations. It is envisaged that such a service would be centred around the already existent Memory Clinic and run by specialist staff adequately trained in the clinical diagnosis and management of dementia and able to provide information on the various aspects of the condition, including disease progression; maintenance of independence; help with memory loss; available support services; treatment options; and financial aspects, as well as contacts to existing dementia societies and support groups. It is believed that investing in early intervention not only improves the quality of life of individuals with dementia and their carers, but is also cost-effective in the long term.

In the various stakeholder consultation meetings, it was evident that early diagnosis and intervention in dementia need to be improved significantly. Carers have expressed their concerns about the lack of advice and appropriate information material at the point of diagnosis. The main impression is that in the majority of cases patients, relatives and carers are left to fend for themselves.

Analysis of the public questionnaire data indicated that a significant number of respondents agreed on the importance of early diagnosis, with more than 90 per cent suggesting the need to diagnose dementia early. Furthermore, more than half of the participants pointed out the significant lack of information on services available to individuals with dementia and their carers (Figure 8.5).

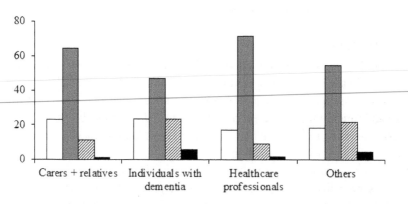

Figure 8.5 Percentage of participants (vertical axis) according to category, indicating whether there is enough information on the services that are available to individuals with dementia and their carers (N/A = not applicable)

A significant number of individuals with dementia and their carers and relatives indicated a certain degree of reluctance to seek medical assistance following the appearance of the first symptoms (Figure 8.6). Approximately 30 per cent of individuals in these categories waited for more than six months before seeking any professional medical advice. Such a time lag can have a negative impact on the pharmacological management of the condition, as the anti-dementia medication currently available is most effective in the early stages of the disease process. The main reasons for eventually seeking medical assistance were problems with memory and difficulties in communication.

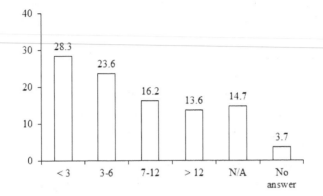

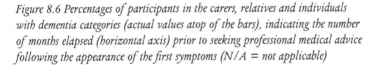

Figure 8.6 Percentages of participants in the carers, relatives and individuals with dementia categories (actual values atop of the bars), indicating the number of months elapsed (horizontal axis) prior to seeking professional medical advice following the appearance of the first symptoms (N/A = not applicable)

Overall, the trends observed showed that dementia in Malta is under-diagnosed and that early intervention needs to be improved considerably. There was an overwhelming agreement on the importance of early diagnosis, as this could lead to postponing residential care and helps individuals with dementia and their carers to take decisions that would enhance their quality of life.

Box 8.2 Recommendations 2 and 3

- *Improve early diagnosis and intervention*
- *Provide good-quality information at the point of diagnosis and beyond*

These recommendations could be achieved by:

1. Promoting and supporting the use of the already existent Memory Clinic in order to receive the load of new dementia cases that is expected to increase in the future. A system whereby a case is followed throughout the course of the disease process should also be developed in order to eliminate the belief that patients and carers are left to manage dementia on their own.

2. Promoting the importance of early diagnosis and intervention in primary care by providing health care professionals with the necessary training and educational tools to diagnose early signs of dementia and provide the necessary advice.

3. Developing an educational pack containing comprehensive good-quality information on the various aspects of dementia and including any available support upon disease disclosure in primary care.

SUPPORT: GOVERNMENT STRUCTURES AND SERVICES

In Malta, elderly people with or without cognitive impairments occupy a significant number of hospital beds. In most cases hospitals are not equipped to provide adequate care to individuals with dementia and lack basic infrastructure, such as proper signage and safety features. Such environments are particularly challenging to individuals with impaired cognitive skills and lead to potentially dangerous situations.

Consultation with stakeholders involved in long-term care indicated that:

1. The number of individuals with dementia is expected to increase in the future and therefore all elderly residential homes need to adopt dementia-friendly design principles.

2. There should be purposely built dementia units to care for patients at different stages of the disease process, and patients should be periodically reassessed during the course of their illness.

3. A system needs to be developed in which residential units housing individuals with dementia are routinely assessed for their standards of care.

4. Due to the nature of the condition, a higher staff–patient ratio was envisaged in care for individuals with dementia. Deployment of human resources should ensure continuity, as constantly changing the staff may be confusing for individuals with dementia.

5. More community services are required in order to reduce early admissions into long-term care. Both health care professionals and the public require an overall change in mentality so that individuals with dementia will not be immediately referred into long-term care.

6. Carers and health care professionals working with dementia patients need to be supported at all levels, to prevent burnout.

The overwhelming majority (85.6%) of individuals participating in the questionnaire, especially among individuals with dementia carers, relatives and health care professionals, agreed on the importance of respite care provision (Figure 8.7).

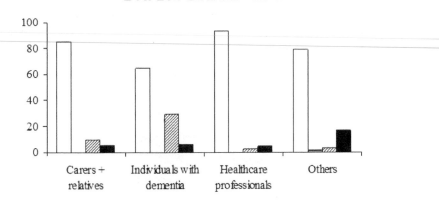

Figure 8.7 Percentage response (vertical axis) by different categories of the Maltese public on the importance of providing respite care (N/A = not applicable)

Although the Memory Clinic has been in use since 2001, only 42 per cent of individuals with dementia, carers and relatives reported that they had made use of this service (Figure 8.8). This was somewhat unexpected, considering the fact that the Memory Clinic is run by health care professionals with specialised training in dementia diagnosis, management and advice. A possible explanation is that this service may be bypassed as a result of diagnosis occurring mainly within primary care.

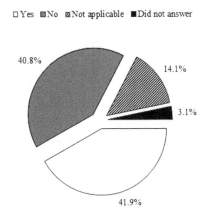

Figure 8.8 Use of the Memory Clinic by individuals with dementia, carers and relatives in Malta

Even though the activity centre at the main state-run elderly residential home provides individuals with dementia with the opportunity of engaging in social interaction through various organised activities and offers the possibility of respite to carers, the service is not very popular. More than half of individuals with dementia and their carers and relatives indicated that they did not use the service (Figure 8.9). The reasons for this may be various and may include the unavailability of organised transport or the belief that proper care can only be provided at home.

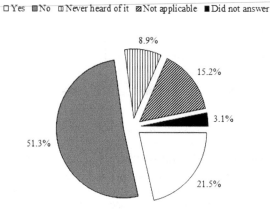

Figure 8.9 The use of the dementia activity centre by individuals with dementia and their carers and relatives

In general there is a need to improve existing public-funded services intended for individuals with dementia and their carers, as well as developing new ways with which these individuals could be assisted. There is a lack of knowledge and information on the availability of specialised services such as the Memory Clinic and activity centres specialising in person-centred dementia care. The lack of financial assistance from central government to support anti-dementia medication, in line with most of the other European countries, also needs to be addressed.

Box 8.3 Recommendations 4, 5 and 6

- *Provide financial support to individuals with dementia in obtaining anti-dementia medication*
- *Increase knowledge on services that are already available for individuals with dementia and their relatives and carers*

- *Improve the quality of care in acute and long-term settings for individuals with dementia, both in state and private medical structures*

These recommendations could be achieved by:

1. The government subsidising anti-dementia medication.

2. Incorporating dementia-friendly design principles in residences accommodating individuals with dementia.

3. Launching an information campaign aimed at informing health care professionals, carers and the general public on the services that are available for individuals with dementia.

4. Increasing the number of activity centres specialising in dementia care, with the possibility of some providing night-time shelter and assistance. Respite care should be available to a wider population of carers and family members.

SUPPORT: COMMUNITY

The majority of individuals with dementia live within the community and most are willing to continue doing so for as long as possible. This is of particular importance in a small country like Malta, in which a significant number of elderly people continue to live with the family. With the right support, these individuals can function effectively within the community, especially in the earliest stages of the condition. As the disease progresses, more services should be available to both the patient and the family carer, thus helping in delaying institutionalisation. It should be ensured that any available or intended new services are reliable and flexible, and have a holistic approach in which decisions about care are taken by health care professionals, the patient and the family.

Currently most of the support available for individuals with dementia and their carers in the community is provided by the Malta Dementia Society and its support group. They regularly organise discussion groups that act as a platform in which carers voice their concerns and share experiences. The benefit of keeping a healthy community network is enormous and should be encouraged in the various possible ways. Due to the psychological burden of caring for individuals with dementia on a daily basis, the need to offer respite care becomes significantly evident. Dementia-specialised activity centres can play an important role in preventing institutionalisation and so allowing patients to live in the community for a longer period of time.

The perceived lack of professional and specialised dementia support in the community was one of the main reasons why the Dementia Strategy Group decided to include a public consultation process as well as seeking feedback from professional stakeholders. Areas that required particular investigation were the importance of community and respite care for individuals with dementia and their carers, as well as the financial strain of dementia caring on the family structure. Such data would be of considerable value for policy makers in the planning of future services intended for individuals with dementia who are still living and being cared for within the community.

Group discussions with stakeholders involved in community care indicated that:

1. Respite care should ideally be available at the patient's residence and in the presence of a trained carer.

2. The provision of good-quality community service will be economically advantageous to the central health authorities and should aid in reducing the current national trend favouring institutionalisation.

3. Psychological support should be available to informal carers in order to assist family members in coping with the stress of dementia care.

4. The home help service should be improved, as currently it is not adequately reaching individuals with dementia.

5. The housing authority needs to be aware of issues related to individuals with dementia, such as safety, access, and arranging for appropriate housing within the community.

6. Members within the community who may be ready to volunteer their time should be involved. The police force should also be trained in dementia awareness as they are among the first-contact categories.

7. There is a need for fast-tracking individuals with dementia and to provide urgent admission and respite when necessary.

8. The carer pension needs to be improved, as the costs involved in caring for individuals with dementia are significantly high.

The majority of respondents among the general public considered community and respite care as significantly important (Figures 8.10, 8.11). Notably, the need of respite was also felt by health care professionals, suggesting that this category is aware that a respite service is a valuable tool for helping informal carers and individuals with dementia to cope with the burden of care. The symptoms that were most difficult to cope with for carers, relatives and individuals with dementia were memory impairments, confusion, and problems with activities of daily living.

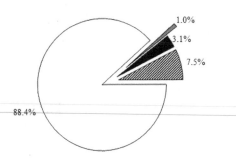

Figure 8.10 *Response from the Maltese public on the importance of community care*

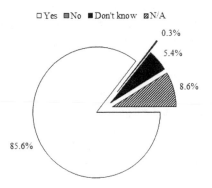

Figure 8.11 *Response from the Maltese public on the importance of respite care*

Caring for an individual with dementia was shown to have a significant impact on family finances. This was expected, as dementia is a costly condition and most of the care provided at home is personally financed by the family. Most of the respondents in the carers, relatives and individuals with dementia categories indicated that they spent more than €100 per month on services related to dementia, with a significant number exceeding €400 per month (Figure 8.12). Most of these expenses go towards private residential and home services and the purchase of anti-dementia medication.

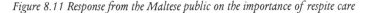

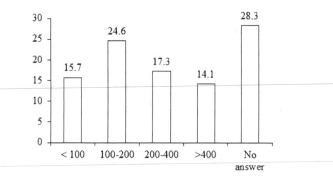

Figure 8.12 Percentage (actual values atop of the bars) of carers, relatives and individuals with dementia spending (in €, horizontal axis) on dementia care per month

Overall, it is clear that community-based dementia services specialised for individuals with dementia and carers are lacking in Malta. Any intervention within the community with the aim of enhancing the quality of life of these individuals will eventually lead to delaying institutionalisation and reduce public spending in the long term. Proper dementia care in residential structures within the community is also lacking due to the absence of dementia-friendly infrastructure and staff trained in patient-centred dementia care. There also needs to be a significant central investment in more activity centres, including respite, for individuals with dementia and their family carers. The financial burden of care within the community also needs to be appropriately addressed.

Box 8.4 Recommendation 7

- *Improve support services for individuals with dementia and their carers within the community*

This recommendation could be achieved by:

1. Developing 'outreach teams' run by health care professionals trained in the medical and social areas of dementia care that will assist individuals with dementia and their carers in the community.

2. Supporting the Malta Dementia Society and the Dementia Helpline in order to be in a better position to assist individuals with dementia and informal carers with good-quality information and advice.

3. Community services offered by the Ministries of Social Services and Health taking into consideration the special needs of individuals with dementia and those who care for them in the community, including financial assistance to purchase new assistive technology

and for any dementia-friendly infrastructural modifications that may be necessary within the patient residential premises.

4. A team of experts in dementia care should be available to routinely monitor and assess government and non-government residential homes accommodating individuals with dementia, in order to ensure that they are of the highest quality and run by adequately trained staff able to offer services that reflect the needs of these individuals.

OTHER ISSUES

End-of-life and palliative care

All across Europe there is a lack of palliative care services for individuals with dementia nearing the final stages of life (Alzheimer Europe 2008). Although these services are routinely offered to terminally ill cancer patients, dementia patients are left out – the main reason being that their condition is not perceived as a terminal illness. It is therefore important that such services should be available to end-stage dementia patients and that the public be informed about the existence of such services. Palliative care also preserves the dignity of the individual and so maximises the quality of life by providing the best level of comfort. It can also offer a support system for family members of the patient to help them cope in their own bereavement.

Almost half of the individuals with dementia and their carers and relatives indicated that end-of-life issues and palliative care are of particular concern (Figure 8.13). This is a significant observation, considering that no such service is available for individuals with dementia in Malta, and so no form of support exists. This continues to highlight the level of psychological stress that family members and carers experience throughout the course of the disease.

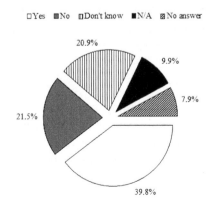

Figure 8.13 Concerns of Maltese individuals with dementia and their carers and relatives about end-of-life issues (N/A = not applicable)

Box 8.5 Recommendation 8

- *Improve end-of-life support services for individuals with dementia and their relatives and carers*

In order to achieve this recommendation, individuals with dementia, health care professionals and carers should be made aware of the need for palliative care in end-stage dementia, and that such a service will enhance the dignity of the individual, as well as being of support to family members. Furthermore, palliative care support already available for end-stage cancer patients in Malta should be available to individuals with dementia and their relatives.

Ethics and legislation

Dementia is a condition that gives rise to various ethical issues for patients, family members and society as a whole (Alzheimer Europe 2010). Legislation in Malta does not make any provision for the needs of individuals with dementia. It is therefore important that both the ethical and legal aspects of the condition are appropriately addressed.

Box 8.6 Recommendation 9

- *Strengthen legal and ethical issues regarding individuals with dementia and their families and carers*

This recommendation can be partly achieved by establishing a group of legal, ethical and dementia-care experts to study in detail the current legal situation in Malta and how it may affect individuals with dementia, and to offer advice on how improvements could be implemented.

Conclusion

Dementia is a condition with lasting consequences for both the patient and the carer. The patient will experience progressive failure of cognitive abilities with time, leading to a significant reduction in ability to function normally as a full member of society. Disease progression will also have a huge impact on the carer, who in most cases is the spouse or a close relative, leading to significant burnout. This is particularly important in countries like Malta where individuals with dementia are mostly cared for within the family structure. This presents important challenges, as the need to offer community support becomes paramount. Unfortunately the results presented in this chapter highlight the lack of awareness and support in many aspects of dementia care in Malta. This was to be expected, considering that mental disorders, especially in close communities, are associated with significant stigma and taboo. It is only in the last few years that discussions on dementia on a national level kicked off, and it would be imprudent to assume that a country with limited resources like Malta could solve such a complex and demanding condition in a short period of time.

Although Malta can become a centre for excellence in dementia care, especially in the research field, where even small interventions can immediately reflect on the whole society, the challenges are not few. It is within the scope of any strategy of this kind to facilitate a shift in public perception of conditions such as dementia. Education and training at any level should be the starting point for addressing this need. Services that support the traditional approach of caring for the elderly should be adapted to include individuals with dementia. Other challenges highlighted by the results presented here include the need for early diagnosis and timely intervention, as these would have a significant impact on quality of life for these patients. The Dementia Strategy Group also recommends an increase in respite care facilities for individuals with dementia living in the community, and the possibility of developing outreach teams that will assist them and their carers at home.

The major challenge would undoubtedly be the financing of such an extended plan, especially in these times of economic crisis across the European continent and beyond. On the other hand, doing nothing is not a real option. Malta has already taken major steps in addressing some important issues in dementia care and the results are evident. The opening of long-term hospital settings specialised in dementia care has not only increased the quality of life of resident individuals with dementia and their carers but is serving as a cornerstone, demonstrating how patient-centred care should be implemented. Such units also serve as a training and education hub for students in the health care professions, giving the opportunity to get hands-on experience in the proper management of dementia. Although such a state-run service is expensive to run, major improvements have already been reported in the quality of care. Such encouraging results would continue to increase momentum in making dementia a top health priority in Malta.

Overall, the various discussions and analysis presented in this chapter emphasise the need to start addressing dementia on a national level, possibly by gradual implementation of the recommendations and suggestions proposed above. These recommendations will not only bring Malta into line with the efforts of other European countries but will also have a huge impact on the quality of life of individuals with dementia, their relatives and carers. The latter are carrying an enormous burden and expect more support from central government and society as a whole. Implementation of these recommendations will also strengthen the current national focus on mental health services for the elderly. It is therefore not surprising that the Maltese health authorities are currently in the process of studying in detail the social and financial implications of these measures in the hope of launching a strategic dementia plan for Malta in the foreseeable future.

References

Abela, S., Mamo, J., Aquilina, C. and Scerri, C. (2007) 'Estimated prevalence of dementia in the Maltese islands.' *Malta Medical Journal 19*, 2, 23–26.

Alzheimer Europe (2008) *End-of-life Care for People with Dementia.* Luxembourg: Alzheimer Europe.

Alzheimer Europe (2010) *Legal Capacity and Proxy Decision Making in Dementia.* Luxembourg: Alzheimer Europe.

Caruana-Pulpan, O. (2010) 'General practioners' approach to diagnosis, disclosure and management of dementia in the Maltese islands.' Master's thesis, University of Malta.

Department for the Elderly and Community Care (2009) *National Dementia Strategy.* Available at https://ehealth.gov.mt/HealthPortal/elderly/dementia/national_dementia_strategy.aspx

Innes, A., Abela, S. and Scerri, C. (2011) 'The organisation of dementia care by families in Malta: the experiences of family caregivers.' *Dementia*, doi:10.1177/1471301211398988

National Statistics Office (2010) *Social Protection: Malta and the EU – Data 2005–2009.* Malta: National Statistics Office.

Scerri, C. and Abela, S. (2006) 'The Malta Dementia Society.' *Journal of the Malta College of Pharmacy Practice 11*, 13–14.

Part III

INNOVATIVE APPROACHES TO CARE

Chapter 9

The Function of Memory Clinics and Post-diagnostic Services for People Newly Diagnosed with Dementia and their Families

Fiona Kelly and Paulina Szymczynska

Introduction

With the rising incidence of dementia in the United Kingdom (UK) (Knapp *et al.* 2007), there is now a political drive to improve services and support to those affected by dementia, including people with dementia themselves, their families and those who work to support them. UK policy on dementia aims to achieve this through ensuring better knowledge about dementia among the general population and those providing support and services, improving early diagnosis, treatment and support for people with dementia and their family members, and improving delivery of services for people's changing needs (Department of Health 2009). There is, crucially, an emphasis on early diagnosis as this is seen to be the gateway for accessing services and support (Department of Health 2009). In a similar focus on the importance of early diagnosis, the Scottish Government has included dementia as one of its core set of health improvement objectives, targets and measures for the National Health Service (NHS), known as HEAT (Health, Efficiency, Access and Treatment) targets (Scottish Government 2007b). This target aims for the early identification and treatment of dementia, and states that 'each NHS Board will achieve agreed improvements in the early diagnosis and management of patients with dementia by March 2011' (Scottish Government 2007b). The target followed the existing national guidance on management of long-term conditions, early intervention to reduce complications, the need for avoidable hospital admission and efficient use of public money (Scottish Executive 2000, 2007a; Scottish Intercollegiate Guidelines Network [SIGN] 2006).

In line with such drivers for early diagnosis (Alzheimer's Foundation of America 2008; Department of Health 2009; Scottish Government 2008), the number of people diagnosed with dementia has been increasing. Connell *et al.* (2009) identified benefits to diagnosis expressed by family members as including obtaining information, having an explanation for the changes noted, and prompting the development of future plans. However, Connell *et al.* also reported barriers to diagnosis, including lack of a cure, the perception by professionals that nothing could be done for the person, and lack of an effective treatment, indicating that more work needs to be done to change public and professionals' perceptions of dementia.

Key policy drivers such as Changing Lives (Scottish Executive 2006) and National Guidance on Self-directed Support (Scottish Government 2007a) have also highlighted the importance of personalisation as a central pillar of the public service reform agenda. Personalisation is defined as an approach that:

> enables the individual alone, or in groups, to find the right solutions for them and to participate in the delivery of a service. From being a recipient of services, citizens can become actively involved in selecting and shaping the services they receive. (Scottish Executive 2007b, p.2)

Personalisation is recognised as a desirable approach to support services for all care groups. If we:

- focus on preventative support, we may reduce the need for more costly support packages designed for crisis – this will have long-term benefits for the system as well as the individual

- devolve more control to individuals and communities and enable people to become participants rather than simply recipients of support, we are more likely to achieve success for individuals first time without having to reinvest in alternatives

- provide individuals with choice and flexibility and a way in which to improve quality, they get the right support at the right time, which has obvious benefits for service provision as well as service users.

(Scottish Executive 2007b)

However, although progress has been made in some fields – for example, in the support of people with learning disabilities – there is little evidence that people with dementia are being offered the opportunity to benefit from self-directed support. The National Guidance (Scottish Executive 2007a) recognises that, although all older people are eligible for self-directed support to meet their assessed personal care needs if they are living at home, currently very few people accessing free personal care do so via self-directed support.

The Changing Lives Service Development Group (Scottish Executive 2006) set out the benefits of personalisation as contributing to: reducing the need for more costly support packages designed for crisis; devolving more control to individuals and communities; and enabling people to become participants rather than simply recipients of support, thus improving the likelihood of achieving success for individuals first time round.

In response to such policy drivers, there have been developments in memory services specialising in the diagnosis of people with dementia and provision of support to them and their families following a diagnosis. This chapter offers useful insight into some of the challenges and opportunities to development and improvement of memory services for people with dementia and their families in rural and urban areas of Scotland.

We will start by introducing the evolution and functions of memory services, specifically memory clinics and post-diagnostic support services. We will then discuss findings from our evaluations of such memory services under the following topic areas: the role of community services; education and training needs of families; and challenges experienced by professionals. We will conclude with a discussion of some implications for practice and some recommendations for service delivery.

Evolution of memory services

In this chapter 'memory services' refers to both memory clinics and post-diagnostic support services – each being potentially complementary to the other in the functions it carries out.

The first memory clinics were set up in the United States in the 1970s and were established in the UK in the 1980s, mainly as academic research centres (Cheung and Strachan 2008; Passmore and Craig 2004). They were set up as dedicated medical interdisciplinary establishments specialising in the assessment and diagnosis of memory disorders (Jolley and Moniz-Cook 2009) and often provided subsequent monitoring of treatment options and patients' progress (Lindesay *et al.* 2002). Professionals most often working in memory clinics include psychologists, consultant psychiatrists, physiotherapists, community psychiatric nurses, team managers and occupational therapists (Alzheimer's Society 2011), although the mix of professionals may vary with locality and resources. The number of memory clinics in the UK has increased in the last two decades, with a corresponding increase in the range of services they offer. According to White (2004), there were approximately 246 memory clinics in the UK in 2004, but there are no official NHS figures and no specific standards or set models allowing monitoring of their development. Key to the Department of Health's (2009) National Dementia Strategy is equity and consistency in pre- and post-diagnostic support and services for people affected by dementia, with acknowledgement that memory clinics are well placed to offer such support.

Memory clinic services in Scotland have been developed to identify and diagnose dementia, develop treatment plans, provide immediate support for people with dementia and family members, and make referrals to appropriate post-diagnostic services, for example the local community mental health team (CMHT), for monitoring and long-term support. In addition to diagnosis, the clinic staff advise patients and families on the meaning of the diagnosis, discuss the importance of power of attorney, driving, financial and welfare benefits, and offer follow-up contact to answer service users' questions and provide emotional support. Memory clinics play a particularly important role in rural areas, where access to specialist services is limited and there is less variability in medical resources (Logan-Sinclair and Davison 2007). Rural memory clinics offer more accessible and efficient service by reducing repeated travel and time to diagnosis, and provision of relevant information about available support (Logan-Sinclair and Davison 2007; Morgan *et al.* 2009).

Following a diagnosis of dementia, people with dementia and their carers should be provided with appropriate support to help them cope, adjust and plan (Department of Health 2009; Leifer 2003). However, they can experience many barriers in the post-diagnostic period, including services not being available in their area (this is particularly relevant in rural areas), lack of awareness of available services, inadequate development of a care plan and lack of communication across services (National Audit Office 2007). Robinson *et al.* (2009) suggest that social service programmes should provide outreach support to carers facing specific stressful conditions (e.g. lack of adequate long-term care services and financial difficulties) and not target those carers who have the support they need. This supports Nolan, Grant and Keady's (1996) suggestion for a more careful targeting of carers who may be at risk of negative health outcomes, rather than a blanket approach that sees all carers (and people with dementia) as being at risk. This would necessitate individual assessments of needs, to take into account not only the challenges experienced, but how these challenges are perceived and the coping strategies employed. The risk with this approach is that some people with dementia and their family members may fall through the gap and be in need of support but unable to access it as a result of not being 'in the system'.

In the urban area, the post-diagnostic service reported on was developed as a model of how to support, enable and empower people with early dementia and their carers, to be able to come to terms with and manage the condition and to take control of the services they need now and in the future. This was a unique service, following the personalisation approach, in which two project staff provided information, advice, signposting and emotional and practical support to people recently diagnosed with dementia and their families, following a referral from local memory clinics. As well as planning ahead, they aimed to support people to find ways to maintain the important relationships in their lives and to remain involved in their communities.

Evaluation of memory services

In the following sections, we present findings from interviews with professionals and practitioners working to support people with dementia and their families via these memory services in rural and urban areas of Scotland.

In the rural area, a consultation with key stakeholders, including people with dementia, family carers and health and social care professionals, was designed to gather information about service structure, range of services provided, challenges and opportunities in dementia practice, and satisfaction with memory services. The consultation processes included a semi-structured questionnaire with ten representatives from community mental health teams (77% response rate) and 20 one-to-one, audio-recorded, semi-structured interviews with seven people with dementia and 13 family carers.

In the urban area, a post-diagnostic memory service was evaluated to explore the difference (or lack of difference) that post-diagnostic support made to people's quality of life in the medium term. Twenty-two professionals and practitioners, including consultant psychiatrists, community mental health teams, physiotherapists, occupational therapists, lawyers, social workers and care managers, were interviewed about their role, current practice and their views and experiences of general post-diagnostic support services provided in the area. We report, specifically, on the views of professionals on the value, difficulties and challenges of delivering post-diagnostic support.

Ethical approval was granted from the local research ethics committees and ethical procedures followed. All interviews were audio-recorded and all audio recordings were transcribed verbatim. Transcripts were read by two researchers to identify initial codes and themes based on the topic guides from interviews and issues arising during the interviews. Analytical themes were arrived at by two researchers following coding and initial analysis, and checked by a third researcher. The role of community services, the importance of carer education and challenges faced by professionals are key areas that affect memory services in rural and urban areas. Each will be discussed in turn.

The role of community services

Community care services have been shown to play a key role in provision of dementia services, including assessment and longer-term support for people with dementia and their carers (Keady, Clarke and Page 2007). The objective of community services is to enable people with dementia to remain at home as long as possible by providing services that address their specific needs (Moriarty and Webb 2000). The main reasons for making referrals to community services are:

- assessment of care needs

- advice on management of problems

- memory assessment

- medical diagnosis.

(Blunden and Long 2002)

Main sources of referrals to community services identified by staff in our evaluations of memory services included general practitioners, social workers and memory clinics. In order to ensure access to diagnostic and post-diagnostic support, the above services need to work together to signpost people with dementia and their carers to appropriate sources of care and support. However, not all people with dementia need community care services. People diagnosed at an early point in their dementia often live independently or rely on family carers and/or service-based support and may not require continuous input from community care services (Page *et al.* 2007). In areas where memory clinic services provide assessment, diagnosis and immediate support, community services have potentially more capacity to focus on providing post-diagnostic support to the clients referred to their service.

Professionals supporting people with dementia and their families in both urban and rural communities reported increasing numbers of people with dementia in their caseloads, with community psychiatric nurse (CPN) services comprising the greatest community support service available in each locality. Notably, dementia cases accounted on average for 64.5 per cent of CPNs' workloads. Similarly, occupational therapy (OT) services reported 64 per cent of their workload dedicated to dementia cases. These findings confirm existing evidence showing the key role of CPNs in providing service users with emotional and practical support (Weaks *et al.* 2009); however, they also indicate a potentially negative consequence, in terms of difficulty in managing workload and sustainability of services, with an ever-increasing caseload of people with dementia and their families.

Findings from our evaluations indicated professionals' commitment to maintaining people at home and revealed the importance of professionals' different roles when providing diagnostic and post-diagnostic services. It was clear that their roles were important in guiding their practice and influencing their experience of service delivery. For some, particularly those giving a diagnosis, a measure of distance between the professional and their patients seems to be important, particularly if they are likely to have to make difficult decisions in the future. Some professionals' roles are, by necessity, task-oriented – for example the OT or physiotherapist looks at the person's functioning ability or safety within the home and will assess for aids or adaptations; the CPN's role is predominantly to monitor and offer support with mental health and particularly to monitor medication; the home care worker will work to support the person with making meals or taking medication in their own home; the social worker will discuss benefits and coordinate services; and a lawyer will offer legal advice or deal with guardianship issues. In many cases professionals referred to each other, indicating good interdisciplinary working, and it was clear from some accounts that a lot of intensive work went into maintaining a person with dementia at home, often involving multidisciplinary team and family input, but also through building up a relationship with a key person over time. There was also some recognition amongst professionals and practitioners that one size does not necessarily fit all, although in practice they continued to refer to generic services such as day centres.

Education and training needs of families

Our findings show that service providers identified the need for education and support courses for people with dementia and their families. In one locality, short courses on dementia were offered and proved to be successful in supporting people with dementia and carers in different aspects of living with dementia. As this was a predominantly rural area, organising centralised group interventions was reported to be difficult. The educational interventions tended to be erratic, due to the unpredictable number of potential participants and limited funding. Therefore the responsibility of educating and supporting service users often lay with those providing community services.

Professionals reported on various ways in which they attempted to meet the educational needs of family members, including one-to-one discussions while visiting them at home, handing out leaflets and holding weekly carer information and support sessions – notably, people with dementia were not included in such sessions. However, our findings suggest that information giving (quality, type, quantity or timing) was, at times, inconsistent and possibly inappropriate and insufficient in some cases. There was the sense among some of the professionals that just giving out information was sufficient, whereas others recognised that this should just be the start in a process that extends over time. However, with the time-limited nature of many of the professionals' roles, this may be difficult if not impossible to achieve.

It was apparent that there was some professional judgement used regarding what information people with dementia and their families needed at particular times, suggesting a more hierarchical than a collaborative approach to information giving. There was also evidence that professionals followed a 'tick box' approach to giving information:

> We're supposed to give everybody certain booklets at certain times and record the fact that we have done. So what this states is that all people who receive dementia diagnosis in the last 12 months should be offered booklets…and the dementia helpline card. (Memory clinic manager)

There was also some recognition, identified more strongly by people with dementia and family members, of differences in support offered to people with Alzheimer's disease as distinct from people with other types of dementia (such as vascular dementia), as this consultant psychiatrist says:

> Most people get a lot of support; if they've got a diagnosis of Alzheimer's disease, they'd see me in the clinic, be given their diagnosis and then be seen [at home by the CPN] on a weekly basis for the first five weeks when they're started on Alzheimer's medication and then followed up at slightly longer intervals. Diagnosis of other conditions (such as vascular dementia) may [involve] less monitoring because there's not such a nursing need to go in because we're not changing medications necessarily. (Consultant psychiatrist)

These findings indicate the desire to provide services and support for people with dementia, but also reveal the discrepancies between what the ideal is and what happens in practice due to resource and time constraints.

Challenges experienced by professionals

Access to diagnostic and post-diagnostic dementia services in rural communities has been argued to be significantly limited (Hansen *et al.* 2005, 2008; Innes *et al.* 2005; Morgan *et al.* 2002; Szymczynska *et al.* 2011). There are a number of barriers to services reported in existing rural research, with the most prominent issues including isolation and distances to specialist services, personal care, residential homes, access to carers' groups, support for the person with dementia, home modifications, disorientating, distressing or inappropriate care and poor relationships with service providers and/or other service users (Hansen *et al.* 2005; Innes, Sherlock and Cox 2003; Innes *et al.* 2005; Morgan *et al.* 2002; Szymczynska *et al.* 2011).

Challenges reported by service providers in rural areas included:

- limited financial and staff resources
- limited transport
- centralised specialist services which are difficult to access
- increasing aging population in the region
- achieving equity in service provision
- stigma and poor awareness of dementia within communities
- diversity of team structures across the region.

These professionals identified three solutions that could potentially aid in overcoming some of the challenges they faced in their practice:

- joint/multiagency working
- minimised bureaucracy
- improved information-sharing (using IT systems and one-to-one communication).

Some of the above challenges can be explained by the diversity of service delivery models across the region. Different team structures and services offered in each locality often make it difficult for staff to communicate and share expertise with colleagues in other teams. Separate IT systems used by health and social care staff do not allow for time- and cost-efficient sharing of important information about patients, lead to duplicated documentation, and result in the need for formal information exchange.

> A good IT system helps to identify work going on, clarifies need, helps establish resources required, enables better working practice in terms of sharing information, etc. (Team leader)

While professionals in urban areas described good interdisciplinary working to provide some excellent post-diagnostic support, including rehabilitation, maintaining the person in the community and monitoring of medication, they also recognised that this support is most often time-limited and goal-oriented. Limited resources and lack of time were cited by these professionals as being key barriers to delivering services effectively to people with dementia and their families. For example, due to time constraints there is limited time to engage in anything other than brief post-diagnostic support or counselling immediately following delivery of a diagnosis; this, to varying degrees, tends to come in the following days, weeks or months.

Lack of resources resulted in some professionals (particularly OTs, physiotherapists and CPNs) having to discharge patients once their condition was stabilised. These professionals were also constrained in the amount and regularity of ongoing post-diagnostic support they could offer. This points to two potential negative consequences for the person with dementia and his or her family. First, the risk of later crisis occurring when the person has been discharged from the particular intervention and has no identified key person monitoring their well-being and/or coping ability. (This applies as much to the carer as the person with dementia.) The second negative consequence is the potential for social isolation if the focus remains only on functional ability, assessment, or medication compliance or monitoring.

Implications and recommendations for service delivery

The process of consulting key stakeholders and sharing the results with them facilitated a bridging of communication between service users, service providers and those commissioning services. This has important implications for the future of dementia services, particularly in the rural area, with a proposed integration of health and social services in this area. Exploring the views of professionals working in memory services also had important implications for service delivery, with findings from questionnaires and service observation allowing development and enhancement of training for dementia care staff (Szymczynska and Innes 2011), facilitating communication of key messages to decision makers and supporting staff to deliver evidence-based support and treatment.

The barriers to use of dementia services in rural and urban communities could potentially be minimised by increased general public awareness of dementia and provision of adequate information and advice. Appropriate interventions should be targeted at combating stigma and encouraging open communication about issues related to dementia in order to obtain support for both people with dementia and their carers. Lack of understanding of various issues related to dementia has been long argued to be the factor affecting service use (Hope, Anderson and Sawyer 2000; Keefover 1996; Kosberg et al. 2004). Health care providers interviewed in Morgan et al.'s (2002) study argued that provision of specific information and advice in the early stages of dementia would lead to increased use of services before crisis situations occur. Regular contact with the health care and community staff has been argued to prevent crisis situations and enable monitoring of support needs, which would diminish the family caregivers' burden and impact on the health system (Morgan et al. 2002).

While this chapter is not specifically focused on people with dementia and their family members, we will include some of their views to illustrate the impact of services and professional input on their everyday experiences and to support recommendations for future services. All those who received post-diagnostic support valued the support offered, and they also spoke about other avenues of support that they found useful. For many, their families and existing friends and networks were invaluable in maintaining social contact and a sense of normality. Some talked of the joy of seeing grandchildren and of the strength of family support, some talked of regular gatherings with long-established friends, others of the golf or bowling club, others of the church. For some people, existing family and networks were most useful in maintaining roles and routine; however, some participants also talked of having to give up certain activities, for example bridge, because of the cognitive difficulties their spouse was experiencing:

> We miss our bridge; we used to play bridge a lot. We don't now, so we both miss that. Well, he was having problems and we just…and it's a very competitive game, it's not like a wee friendly game of cards, it's not just a wee friendly night out, it's a serious thing, and they're picking winners and things like that. But it's…you get the feeling you're spoiling other people's game, if you're not quite 100 per cent, so we've just…just didn't go back. (Carer)

Others talked of friends dropping away, either because they were ill, had died or were unable to cope with the diagnosis. One participant stopped going to church because she was unable to understand the service, thereby losing a whole network of people. These examples indicate the potential for supportive networks to decline and the importance of having other mechanisms in place to take over when that happens.

Although there was positive feedback on usual services, particularly the response to crises, many people, particularly those with vascular or mixed dementia, had little or no regular contact with memory services:

> No follow-up appointments, no. No. In fact, I was just thinking I'll wait until near the beginning of the year, and it'll be nearly two years, and then I'll make an appointment to see Doctor X again, because I think after two years we definitely should be seeing somebody, do you not agree? (Carer)

> She [consultant psychiatrist] explained what vascular dementia was. That's all I remember about her visiting there. And would this have been within the last six months or like over a year ago? I'm thinking a year, maybe longer; it could be two years. (Carer)

Two participants noted that the initial, more intensive support from the memory clinic has since stopped:

> Yes, it [initial support] is good and then it just stops. If you need them, phone them. That's all. That's it. Nobody pops in, you know, you're kind of just left on your own. To get on with it!... I just feel that once you have been diagnosed you have got no...you know, they don't have any contact with you. They don't...there's nothing. What's the word? There's no aftercare. (Carer)

These accounts illustrate the importance of people's family and networks as sources of support. However, for various reasons these may decline or disappear altogether, leaving the person with dementia and their carer at risk of isolation. As memory clinics and other health services are constrained in the amount and regularity of ongoing post-diagnostic support they can offer, and as, in many cases, the level of support drops off once the person with dementia is stable (medication or functioning), post-diagnostic services have the potential to fill possible gaps (declining networks, reducing clinical input) and can offer ongoing, longer-term support, whether through social events, advice, information and help with planning ahead as needed and wished.

Conclusion

The timing of support provision, both in terms of diagnosing dementia in its early stages and of offering early intervention and ongoing support following a diagnosis, can be key to empowering individuals to remain in their homes for as long as appropriate and avoiding crisis situations. While memory clinics have the potential to address the need for accessible diagnostic services, they need to work jointly with other services providing post-diagnostic care, to ensure that individuals newly diagnosed with dementia and their families have stable access to required care and support throughout the progression of dementia. However, with the increasing rates of referrals to post-diagnostic services, service providers are under pressure to deliver best quality care with the limited resources that are available.

The findings about memory services reported in this chapter illustrate the issues shared by service providers in urban and rural areas. Limited availability of services and resources presents a significant obstacle to provision of appropriate care and support for people with a diagnosis of dementia and their family carers. Although staff make efforts to follow best practice evidence and good standards of care, the limited resources and the obligation to adhere to set procedures often mean that they have to neglect their own judgement, be selective in following a person-centred approach, and forgo developing innovative approaches to care.

There seems to be a dual drive toward increasing the efficiency of services through introducing sets of procedures and task-oriented roles, and following good practice advocating a person-centred approach, taking innovative approaches to care and carrying out ongoing monitoring of patients. It is unlikely that the availability of resources will improve in the near future; therefore the way services are delivered to people with dementia and their families will have to be reconsidered to achieve a balance between the cost of dementia care and its quality.

Acknowledgements

Thank you to Anthea Innes, Cameron Stark, Lynda Forrest and Sherry Macintosh for their roles in the research that has informed this chapter. Thank you, also, to the participants who gave their time to tell us of their experiences of memory services.

References

Alzheimer's Foundation of America (2008) *Memory Matters: Screening Approaches to Increase Early Detection and Treatment of Alzheimer's Disease and Related Dementias, and recommendations for National Policy.* New York: AFA.

Alzheimer's Society (2011) *Diagnosis and Assessment.* Available at www.alzheimers.org.uk/site/scripts/documents_info.php?documentID=260

Blunden, P. and Long, R. (2002) 'Dementia and GP referrals to CPNs.' *Mental Health Nursing 22,* 4, 8–12.

Cheung, G. and Strachan, J. (2008) 'A survey of memory clinics in New Zealand.' *Australian Psychiatry 16,* 4, 244–247.

Connell, C., Roberts, J., McLaughlin, S. and Carpenter, B. (2009) 'Black and white adult family members' attitudes toward a dementia diagnosis.' *Journal of the American Geriatrics Society 57,* 9, 1562–1568.

Department of Health (2009) *Living Well with Dementia: A National Dementia Strategy.* London: Department of Health. Available at www.iow.nhs.uk/uploads/General/pdfs/Living%20well%20with%20dementia%20-%20a%20National%20Dementia%20Strategy%20-%20Accessible%20Summary.pdf

Hansen, E., Robinson, A., Mudge, P. and Crack, G. (2005) 'Barriers to the provision of care for people with dementia and their carers in a rural community.' *Australian Journal of Primary Health 11,* 1, 72–79.

Hansen, E.C., Hughes, C., Routley, G. and Robinson, A.L. (2008) 'General practitioners' experiences and understanding of diagnosing dementia: factors impacting on early diagnosis.' *Social Science and Medicine 67,* 11, 1776–1783.

Hope, S., Anderson, S. and Sawyer, B. (2000) *The Quality of Services in Rural Scotland.* Edinburgh: The Stationery Office, Scottish Executive Central Research Unit.

Innes, A., Sherlock, K. and Cox, S. (2003) 'Seeking the views of people with dementia on services in rural areas.' *Journal of Dementia Care 11,* 5, 37–38.

Innes, A., Sherlock, K., Smith, A., Mason, A. and Cox, S. (2005) 'Dementia care provision in rural Scotland: service users' and carers' experiences.' *Health and Social Care in the Community 13,* 4, 354–365.

Jolley, D. and Moniz-Cook, E. (2009) 'Memory clinics in context.' *Indian Journal of Psychiatry 51,* S70–76.

Keady, J., Clarke, C. and Page, S. (2007) *Partnerships in Community Mental Health Nursing and Dementia Care: Practice Perspectives.* Maidenhead: Open University Press.

Keefover, R. (1996) 'The clinical epidemiology of Alzheimer's disease.' *Neurology Clinics 14,* 2, 337–351.

Knapp, M., Prince, M., Albanese, E., Banerjee, S. *et al.* (2007) *Dementia UK.* London: Alzheimer's Society.

Kosberg, J., Leeper, J., Burgio, L. and Kaufman, A. (2004) 'Family caregivers of aged persons with dementia living in rural Alabama.' [Abstract.] In the Gerontological Society of America 57th Annual Scientific Meeting, 19–23 November, Washington DC. *The Gerontologist 44* (Special Issue I), 110.

Leifer, B.P. (2003) 'Early diagnosis of Alzheimer's disease: Clinical and economic benefits.' *Journal of the American Geriatrics Society 51,* 5, S281–S288.

Lindesay, J., Marudkar, M., va Diepen, E. and Wilcock, G. (2002) 'The second Leicester survey of memory clinics in the British Isles.' *International Journal of Geriatric Psychiatry 17*, 1, 41–47.

Logan-Sinclair, P.A. and Davison, A. (2007) 'Diagnosing dementia in rural New South Wales.' *Australian Journal of Rural Health 15*, 183–188.

Morgan, D.G., Crossley, M., Kirk, A., D'Arcy, C. *et al.* (2009) 'Improving access to dementia care: development and evaluation of a rural and remote memory clinic.' *Aging and Mental Health 13*, 1, 17–30.

Morgan, D.G., Semchuk, K.M., Stewart, N.J. and D'Arcy, C. (2002) 'Rural families caring for a relative with dementia: barriers to use of formal services.' *Social Sciences and Medicine 55*, 7, 1129–1142.

Moriarty, J. and Webb, S. (2000) *Part of their Lives: Community Care for Older People with Dementia.* Bristol: The Policy Press.

National Audit Office (2007) *Improving Services and Support for People with Dementia.* London: The Stationery Office.

Nolan, M., Grant, G. and Keady, J. (1996) *Understanding Family Care.* Buckingham: Open University Press.

Page, S., Hope, K., Bee, P. and Burns, A. (2007) 'Nurses making a diagnosis of dementia – a potential change in practice?' *International Journal of Geriatric Psychiatry 23*, 1, 27–33.

Passmore, A.P. and Craig, D.A. (2004) 'The future of memory clinics.' *Psychiatric Bulletin 28*, 10, 375–377.

Robinson, J., Fortinsky, R., Kleppinger, A., Shugrue, N. and Porter, M. (2009) 'A broader view of family caregiving: effects of caregiving and caregiver conditions on depressive symptoms, health, work and social isolation.' *Journal of Gerontology Social Sciences 64B*, 6, 788–798.

Scottish Executive (2000) *Fair Shares for All: Final Report.* Available at www.scotland.gov.uk/Topics/Health/care/FairShares/FullReport [accessed 10 May 2011].

Scottish Executive (2006) *Changing Lives.* Report of the 21st Century Social Work Review. Edinburgh: Scottish Executive.

Scottish Executive (2007a) *All Our Futures: Planning for a Scotland with an Ageing Population.* Available at www.scotland.gov.uk/Topics/People/Equality/18501/Experience [accessed 10 May 2011].

Scottish Executive (2007b) *Personalisation: An Agreed Understanding.* Changing Lives Service Development Group. Edinburgh: Scottish Executive. Available at www.socialworkscotland.org.uk/resources/private/Personalisation.pdf [accessed 18 February 2011].

Scottish Government (2007a) *National Guidance on Self-directed Support.* Edinburgh: Scottish Government.

Scottish Government (2007b) *HEAT Targets.* Available at www.scotland.gov.uk/Topics/Health/NHS-Scotland/17273/targets [accessed 10 May 2011].

Scottish Government (2008) *HEAT Targets.* Available at www.scotland.gov.uk/Topics/Health/mental-health/servicespolicy/DFMH/antidepressantprescribing [accessed 3 January 2012].

Scottish Intercollegiate Guidelines Network (2006) *Management of Patients with Dementia: A National Clinical Guideline.* Edinburgh: SIGN.

Szymczynska, P. and Innes, A. (2011) 'Evaluation of a dementia training workshop for health and social care staff in rural Scotland.' *Remote and Rural Health Journal 11*, 2, 1611.

Szymczynska, P., Innes, A., Mason, A. and Stark, C. (2011) 'A review of diagnostic process and post-diagnostic support for people with dementia in rural areas.' *Journal of Primary Care and Community Health 2*, 4, 262–276.

Weaks, D., Johansen, R., Wilkinson, H. and McLeod, J. (2009) *'There is Much More to My Practice than Checking up on Tablets.' Developing Nursing Practice: A Counselling Approach to Delivering Post-Diagnostic Dementia Support.* Edinburgh: University of Edinburgh.

White, E. (2004) 'Memory clinics can make a difference.' *Mental Health Nursing 25*, 3, 18–19.

Chapter 10

Bridging the Gap for Dementia Care in India

Amit Dias

Dementia amidst the demographic transition in India

India is emerging as a strong, self-reliant, modern nation. The country occupies only 2.4 per cent of the world's surface area but is home to one sixth of the world's population. With improving health care, life expectancy is on the rise and the country is going through rapid demographic transition. As a result we expect to see a larger burden of chronic diseases such as dementia in India. The Dementia India Report released in 2010 (Alzheimer's and Related Disorders Society of India [ARDSI] 2010) estimated that there were around 3.7 million people with dementia in India, and that the numbers were set to double by the year 2030 (ARDSI 2010). Alzheimer's disease is the fourth leading cause of death compared to other chronic medical conditions in the Asian Pacific region (Alzheimer's Disease International 2006). The 10/66 dementia research group has engaged in a number of epidemiological studies in India and other low and middle income countries to reveal the hidden epidemic and find possible solutions to bridge the wide treatment gap in these regions (see Box 10.1).

Box 10.1 The 10/66 dementia research group

The 10/66 dementia research group derives its name from the fact that only 10 per cent of the total research on dementia is directed towards the 66 per cent or more of all people with dementia who live in developing countries. 10/66 was founded in India in 1998 and is now the official research wing for Alzheimer's Disease International, UK. Over 100 active researchers from over 30 developing countries form a part of this network. More information is available at www.alz.co.uk/10/66-group.

Care for people with dementia in India

Families: the sole source of support

India is a country known for its traditional values and rich cultural heritage. Families are still the main source of care for people with dementia in India. However, they are now finding it difficult to cope with the demands of a person with dementia due to the changing scenario, as the traditional joint family system where the members felt it was their bounden duty to care for the elderly and disabled in the family slowly breaks up. Nuclear families or three-generation families (where the parents live with their son's family) are the new norm (ARDSI 2010; NISD 2008). Often the children are working overseas and their parents stay back home without much support (see Case study 10.1). Women, who traditionally played the role of homemakers, are now employed to cope with increasing demands in life. Given this situation, it is slowly becoming difficult for family members to cope with the increasing demands of caring for older people even if they wish to do so, leaving them helpless (ARDSI 2010). This predicament is clearly illustrated in Case study 10.2 which is a common scenario resulting from the changing family structure in this country. It is also noticed that caregivers of people with dementia are often unaware of the diagnosis, and so do not understand the changed behaviours that accompany this condition. As in most cultures, almost 80 per cent of caregivers are females and 50 per cent are spouses who themselves are over the age of 60 years (Dias *et al.* 2004; 10/66 DRG 2004).

Case study 10.1 Susheela makes tea for her joint family

Susheela lived in a joint family with 13 members. She used to handle the cooking for all the family members. She lost her husband a few years ago and her children migrated abroad for better prospects. She now lives alone with a maid. The maid brought her to our clinic saying that Susheela is quite forgetful and will go to the kitchen and make tea for 13 people.

Case study 10.2 Sushmita stretched between two families

Sushmita lives in California. Her father, who lives in India, had a stroke and was later diagnosed as having vascular dementia. He was looked after by Sushmita's mother. Everything was fine until her mother passed away a few months ago. Now he has been moved to Sushmita's brother's house. However, her brother's wife threatened to leave the house if Sushmita's father continues to live with them. Sushmita says that she is stretched between her family commitments and love for her father with a chronic illness.

Organizations providing dementia support

In 1992 the Alzheimer's and Related Disorders Society of India (ARDSI) was established as a not-for-profit organization in response to the need for care and support for people with dementia and their families. It was established under the leadership of Dr K. Jacob Roy, a paediatrician by profession, who had a personal encounter with the condition when his father began to show signs of Alzheimer's disease. Today ARDSI has several chapters in the country and intends to expand further. ARDSI represents the voice of people with dementia and their caregivers in India and is making an attempt to get dementia on the public health agenda of the country. ARDSI firmly believes that a dementia-friendly state can only be established if there is political and social commitment at all levels. Besides ARDSI, some other organizations have also started extending support to people with dementia in the country – for example, the Dementia Society of Goa, Sangath, Nightingales Trust, Dignity Foundation, Silver Innings, and a few others.

Specialized dementia services

There are a number of residential homes for the elderly in India; however, they selectively refuse to admit people with dementia as they find it difficult to cope with an individual who is likely to have problem behaviours, due to lack of trained staff. It is only recently that a few specialized residential homes and day-care centres have emerged as a response to the growing awareness drive by ARDSI. According to the Dementia India Report released by ARDSI in 2010 (ARDSI 2010), there were just six residential care facilities and ten day-care centres for people with dementia in the country, which is grossly inadequate considering the huge size of the population in this country.

There are over 100 memory clinics in the country providing diagnostic services and other services. Memory clinics are used for evaluating people with memory complaints and providing medication if necessary. Post-diagnostic support is also provided to the caregiver and the person with dementia. As of now in 2011, almost two-thirds of the memory clinics are supported by pharmaceutical companies. The pharmaceutical companies do it as part of their corporate social responsibility, but the move is mutually beneficial as more dementia-specific medications will be prescribed once a diagnosis is made. All drugs specific for the management of dementia are available in India. Almost all super-speciality hospitals with psychiatry or neurology services have memory clinics. However, in contrast, very few of the other medical hospitals have such services, resulting in the vast majority of the population being denied access to basic diagnostic facilities for dementia.

Impact on caregivers of people with dementia

Studies carried out in India revealed that caring for people with dementia was associated with increased physical, mental and financial strain on the caregiver (Dias *et al.* 2004; 10/66 DRG 2004). Studies have also shown that the levels of caregiver strain in low and middle income countries are comparable to those in the European EUROCARE project (10/66 DRG 2004; Prince *et al.* 2009). Around 60 per cent of the 179 caregivers enrolled in the Indian 10/66 study showed adverse mental health impact, as recorded by the general health questionnaire used in the study for this purpose (10/66 DRG 2004). However, we did come across some caregivers who looked at their role as an opportunity to serve their loved ones. Case studies 10.3 and 10.4 are examples of how different caregivers may react to similar situations in completely different ways. The positive outlook towards care has a lot to do with cultural and religious factors. Caregiving sometimes gives a person a sense of identity, and they would leave no stone unturned to do a good job, which is very fortunate for the person in their care. However, such situations are very rare. 'My husband always remembered to buy me a gift for my birthday…now he does not remember me,' says Margarita, who has been looking after her husband diagnosed with Alzheimer's disease for the last ten years. 'I love him and he loves me, and that is all that matters,' she adds tearfully.

CASE STUDY **10.3** CAREGIVER BURNOUT

Akshata, who is a working mother, found it difficult to understand why her mother-in-law was suddenly accusing her of keeping her hungry and would get into an argument over petty issues. Her mother-in-law would not have a bath, and when she was told to do so she would insist that she was clean and had had a shower. Unknown to Akshata, her mother-in-law had early signs of dementia. Akshata found it very difficult to look after her two small children and her mother-in-law, who she felt was getting stubborn and increasingly difficult to handle. With little help from her husband, who was working overseas, she admitted that she often felt that life was not worth living.

CASE STUDY **10.4** CAREGIVING AS A DIVINE OPPORTUNITY

Maria is a housewife and is also looking after her mother-in-law who has dementia. Her mother-in-law is dependent on her for food and almost all activities of daily living. She also gets violent at times, but cools down like a lamb the very next moment, Maria describes. 'Ever since I started looking after my mother-in-law, my health has improved,' she says. Maria has come to terms with her role as a caregiver and feels that there is a divine plan for all that happens.

Health-seeking behaviour and the cost of care

Several community-based studies have shown that people with dementia prefer services provided by private doctors (Dias *et al.* 2004; 10/66 DRG 2004). This is mainly because private doctors provide home visits, which families find more convenient compared to taking the person with dementia to a government health facility, where there are often long queues. A publication by the 10/66 dementia research group reveals that, of the 179 people with dementia studied, 56 per cent had visited a private doctor, 5 per cent visited a government primary care and government hospital, 11 per cent required hospital admissions and 1 per cent visited traditional healers, while 33 per cent did not visit any health facility (10/66 DRG 2004). Visits to the health facility, however, were not specifically on account of the memory problem.

The fact that private doctors are preferred also explains why the medical cost of caring for a person with dementia is considerably higher than that of caring for elders with other chronic illnesses. The primary health care system does not have the option of providing home visits by doctors, but it does have multi-purpose health workers who visit the community in the region assigned to them. However, these local health functionaries lack the skills necessary to provide support for families of people with dementia. The Dementia India Report (2010) estimates the total societal cost of caring for all people with dementia in India is INR 147 billion (US$ 3.4 billion) if basic care were to be provided for people with dementia (ARDSI 2010). However, calculating the economic impact of dementia is a complex task and requires further research in developing countries, as very little information is available.

The wide treatment gap for dementia

The 'treatment gap' for dementia indicates the difference between the total number of people with dementia and those people with dementia who receive at least basic, evidence-based care. In a study conducted in Goa (Dias *et al.*

2008), in which 81 people with dementia participated, only 5 per cent (4) had received a diagnosis and treatment specific for dementia. This is despite the fact that 51 per cent (41) had been seen by a physician in the previous three months. This amounts to a treatment gap of over 90 per cent, even in the relatively prosperous state of Goa which has much better health facilities compared to the rest of the states in the country. The Dementia India Report refers to a similar treatment gap across the whole country (ARDSI 2010). The Goa study also revealed that some families refused to accept dementia-specific medications, indicating reasons such as high costs, fear of side effects, and the family physician advising them against it.

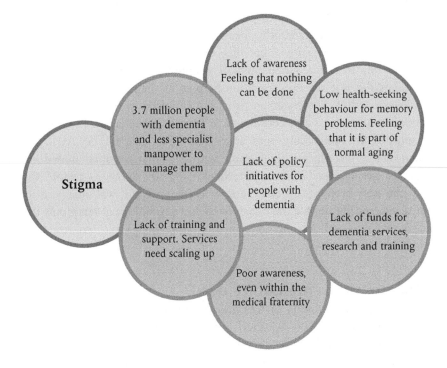

Figure 10.1 Barriers to dementia care

There are several major barriers to closing this treatment gap for dementia, as illustrated in Figure 10.1. These include the low levels of awareness, the huge burden in terms of numbers of people with dementia in the country, and stigma associated with behavioural problems accompanying the condition. However, the most significant barrier is the low human resource capacity for care of people with dementia and this, once again, is due to the large number of people with dementia in the country. The scarcity of resources is true for the whole spectrum of mental disorders. This has been systematically documented in the recent *Lancet* series on global mental health (Saxena *et al.* 2007). India, like most of the low and middle income countries, lacks the economic and social capital to achieve widespread coverage of specialist services (Prince *et al.* 2009). It is necessary to find a way to overcome these barriers, using locally available resources, in order to reach out to people with dementia (Dias and Patel 2009).

Help-seeking behaviour for people with dementia

Memory problems in older people are generally considered part of normal aging (ARDSI 2010; Patel and Prince 2001). A study conducted in Goa assessed the knowledge, attitudes and practices regarding dementia, and revealed that caregivers and other health care providers recognized the signs and symptoms of dementia – but they didn't consider that it was a health problem, nor that it required medical attention; the primary health care physicians did not see this condition as part of their clinical work (Patel and Prince 2001). There was no name for dementia in the local language, as traditionally it was not considered to be a separate entity. (This is true for most of the Indian languages, apart from a few; see ARDSI 2010. The fallout of this ignorance is that people with dementia are often abused and neglected; see Patel and Prince 2001; Shaji *et al.* 2002.) Very few people with dementia were brought to a clinic, and when they were, it was usually in the late stages, specifically for the behavioural and psychological symptoms that accompany the condition and not primarily for memory loss (Ferri, Ames and Prince 2004).

What does the community need?

The challenge for a country such as India is to develop culturally appropriate interventions that can be delivered using existing resources. Planning for service development in India should keep in mind that services should be home-based, address the diverse medical and psychological needs of people with dementia and their caregivers, and be provided at a cost that the family can afford, by using the existing primary health care system which is provided by the government free of cost.

The Dementia Home Care Project: a response to the need

The Dementia Society of Goa developed an intervention in response to the complex needs of people with dementia and their families using locally available resources (Dias *et al.* 2008). The interventions were delivered in a flexible, stepped care model. This means that frequent visits and more intense intervention was provided to those who needed it the most (e.g. caregivers of people with dementia who also had behavioural problems or who needed more support with regard to the activities of daily living). What was unique about this project was that the intervention was provided by home care advisors (HCAs) who were non-specialist workers under the supervision of a psychiatrist and a counsellor. The only qualification for the HCA was that he/she had to be literate, know the local language, preferably have passed higher secondary school, and be motivated to do work in the community.

The HCAs were trained for a week to help them gain specific knowledge and skills, such as listening and counselling skills, understanding dementia and the non-pharmacological management of psychological and behavioural problems that accompany the condition, and assisting with activities of daily living and the management of common health problems in older people. Repeated refresher training programmes were also held for them.

Design of the intervention

The intervention focused on the use of non-specialist health workers for providing support to families of people with dementia. It was evaluated using a randomized controlled trial – a design often used to test new drugs in the market. A total of 81 dyads of people with dementia and their caregivers were recruited into the trial. The intervention was randomly provided for six months to one group of individuals and it was compared with the effects of usual care received by the group allocated to the control arm. The HCAs were supervised by a counsellor and psychiatrist who would meet them every fortnight to discuss the cases and develop a protocol for the intervention. The intervention followed a flexible, stepped care model where all families were visited once every fortnight; however, those families that required more care were given more frequent visits. For example, caregivers who were older or were looking after people with a lot of behavioural problems were more likely to be suffering burnout, and so would be given more frequent visits.

Interventions under the Home Care Programme

Since the interventions were provided by non-specialist workers, there was a lot of emphasis on their training and supervision. The training module was divided into ten sections to cover various interventions for the person with dementia as well as the caregiver, as enumerated below.

1. Identify stress in the caregivers

The HCAs help the caregivers to make time for themselves and to learn the art of congratulating themselves if no one else does. 'It's been six years since I am looking after Edmund and no one appreciated what I did till you came by,' said one caregiver to our HCA. The HCAs would encourage other family members to express their appreciation towards the caregiver.

2. Balance family support

Quite often it was noticed that the person with dementia was looked after by one family member and their role was taken for granted. The primary caregiver also had to do the shopping and cooking and pay the bills. The HCAs would try to understand the situations and encourage the other family members to do some of the activities, even if it was not directly looking after the person with dementia.

3. Help the family understand dementia

Understanding the condition is key to understanding its management and understanding the behaviour of the person. The HCAs were trained to help the family understand that life does not end with the diagnosis of dementia and that a lot can be done to improve the quality of life of the person with dementia. With the availability of the internet, some of the family members might read about the condition, but the information might not reach the primary caregiver, who may not have access to such material.

4. Understand behavioural problems associated with dementia

Caregivers found the behavioural problems associated with the condition most distressing, and often this was the first complaint that brought them in desperation to a clinic. Behavioural problems are associated with a lot of stigma. The HCA would assess the behavioural problems in the person with dementia, using a structured questionnaire, and would advise simple, non-pharmacological means of addressing them. For example, they would train the caregiver in how to deal with repeated questioning by distracting the person or giving them written answers to frequently asked questions. They would try to help the caregiver understand any trigger for violent behaviour, screaming episodes or hallucinations, and find solutions to address them. The HCAs would discuss the problem with the counsellor and psychiatrist on their regular visits and decide the best course of action.

5. Assisting activities of daily living

The HCAs assessed the functional ability of the person with dementia and would help the caregivers with simple techniques to assist them with activities of daily living. The activities of daily living were assessed using structured questionnaires, and the caregivers would be encouraged to help the person maintain functioning as far as possible. For example, the person with dementia would be encouraged to manage activities of daily living independently – eat, shower, dress, etc. The HCAs would identify the activities that were easily performed and those to which there was resistance, and the time of the day when it happened. Often the problem behaviours were more frequently encountered in the evening, and the caregivers were encouraged to do all their work with the person with dementia in the morning, when they were much more cooperative. This was done to try and help the person with dementia maintain their independence and functioning for longer.

6. Making the home safe for people with dementia

A cluttered home environment can confuse a person with dementia, and at the same time make it unsafe for the person. The HCAs would help the family to identify situations that could be a possible threat, and help them to change the environment and keep harmful items out of reach (see Case study 10.5).

Case study 10.5 Safety is essential

Catherina, a person with dementia, looked as if she was making tea when the home care advisor first visited her house. On taking a closer look the HCA realized that Catherina was mixing tea leaves in cold water. The HCA also smelt cooking gas (fuel) in the house. She realized that Catherina was alone, and trying to prepare tea; she had managed to switch on the gas but could not find the matchbox. Had she found it, the whole house could have gone up in flames.

Threats to life can be all over the house – a floor detergent that looks like milk, medications, kitchen appliances, sharp items, hot water in the shower, stairs, windows without grills, slippery floors, doormats and other items that can lead to falls... The HCAs would inspect the house with the caregiver to identify potential causes of harm and place them out of reach.

7. Structuring the day

The HCAs would help the caregivers to structure the day and maintain a daily schedule for activities. For example, they would help the caregiver decide what should be done in the morning, afternoon, evening and at night. This was mainly based on the person's previous routine. In this manner they would gain cooperation from the person with dementia to carry out activities of daily living. Quite often the person with dementia would be served food at times most convenient for the caregiver – sometimes before and sometimes after all the other family members had eaten. This would disturb the routine and lead to resistance while eating. The HCAs would try to identify those parts of the day when the person with dementia was most receptive to suggestions, so as to get most of the necessary work completed in that period.

8. Medical management

Some of the people with dementia were suitable candidates for medical management, and they were encouraged to carry on with their medication. They were encouraged to meet the psychiatrist on the project at least once during the intervention. A home visit by the psychiatrist was arranged if a clinic visit was not possible. The rest of the follow-up was done by the HCAs.

9. Advice on additional medical conditions

Some people with dementia also had other medical conditions, such as diabetes and hypertension. These were often neglected after the onset of dementia. The family and, wherever possible, the person with dementia were encouraged to continue with their medication for additional medical ailments. Appropriate advice on other non-pharmacological management, such as nutrition, was given in consultation with the experts.

10. Developing a support system

A helpline was created for assisting the family members supporting a relative with dementia. The programme helped in initiating self-help support groups. However, it was not possible to sustain this initiative, as quite often the primary caregivers could not attend meetings because they were unable to find even a short-term substitute to take over their role. They also had problems with transport to attend meetings.

The interventions were evaluated at baseline and every three months for a total of six months by researchers who remained blinded to (unaware of) the intervention status. Standardized and validated instruments such as the General Health Questionnaire (GHQ), Zarit Burden Scale (ZBS; Zarit, Reeve and Bach-Paterson 1980), Neuro Psychiatric Inventory Questionnaire (NPIQ; Cummings *et al.* 1994) and Everyday Ability Scale for India (EASI; Fillenbaum, Chandra and Ganguli 1999) were used to evaluate caregiver stress, perceived burden, impact of behavioural problems, and functional ability of the person with dementia.

Results of the interventions demonstrated a significant impact in reducing the perceived caregiver burden, mental stress, and distress due to behavioural and psychological symptoms of dementia. It also showed a non-significant reduction in the total number of deaths of people with dementia in the intervention arm, which could indicate an improvement in the quality of their life. There was, however, no significant improvement in the functional ability of the person with dementia.

The programme demonstrates that it is possible to introduce a community dementia outreach programme as part of the existing primary health care set-up, relying on trained non-specialist community health workers supervised by mental health (or other appropriately trained) specialists. This is possibly the cost-effective solution to bridge the treatment gap in the country. The intervention won the Fondation Médéric Alzheimer and the Alzheimer Disease International prize for being the best evidence-based psychosocial intervention for families of people with dementia in 2010.

Reaching out and closing the treatment gap for dementia

In an attempt to find possible solutions to the growing public health concern in the country, ARDSI took the initiative of organizing consultative meetings of experts, doing a systematic review of the research carried out on dementia in the country and developing the Dementia India Report. The expert committee also studied dementia policies from other parts of the developed world to come up with core areas that India needs to focus on in the coming years. They identified seven core areas that need to be addressed in order to develop and deliver services to the community at large (see Table 10.1).

Table 10.1 Seven core strategies for delivering dementia care services

What to deliver	How to deliver	Who could deliver	Where to deliver
1. Raise awareness and create a demand for services.	Effective use of media and films, provide disability benefits to people with dementia and caregivers, fight stigma, improve quality and accessibility of services.	Government, not-for-profit organizations, health professionals, media.	Community, primary care, memory clinics.
2. Capacity building of health care teams.	Training medical nursing fraternity in dementia management, train health care workers, Anganwadi[1] workers and ASHA[2] in delivering long-term care.	Doctors, nurses, multipurpose health workers, ASHA[2] and other community outreach workers (non-specialist health care volunteers).	Hospitals, including primary health care centres.
3. Provide affordable treatment (pharmacological and psychological).	Develop and use cheaper generic versions of anti-dementia drugs. Use existing resources for care. Integrate long-term care and support interventions into programmes for all dependent elderly.	Patients on anti-dementia drugs can be followed up by the primary care physicians after being seen by a specialist. Community health workers could be trained in long-term care.	Community primary health care level.

4. Effective long-term care through community-based programmes.	Train carers to establish support groups, domiciliary visits to families of people with dementia.	Community health workers, or staff specially appointed for community elder care.	Primary care, community.
5. Residential, respite and day care facilities.	Specialized facilities with trained personnel could be established for this purpose. This will cater to the severe cases of dementia or those who do not have any support.	Not-for-profit organizations, government.	Community.
6. Develop legal services.	Provide the much-needed legal support.	Not-for-profit organizations, government, law-enforcement agencies.	Community.
7. Develop training services.	Institutes for training geriatric home nurses. Training workshops for medical fraternity could be established.	Government, not-for-profit organizations.	Throughout the country.

Source: adapted with permission from the Dementia India Report

1   Anganwadi worker: local health functionaries under the Integrated Child Development Services (ICDS) scheme.
2   Accredited Social Health Activists (ASHA): local health functionaries under the National Rural Health Mission.

The World Health Organization (WHO) suggests that, in view of the rapid demographic transition in developing countries, it is necessary to enact what they term 'active aging' policies and programmes that enhance the health, independence and productivity of older citizens (WHO 2002). The WHO has recently launched the Mental Health Gap Action Programme (mhGAP) specifically to look at the gap in services for conditions affecting mental health. It lists dementia as one of the major priorities and makes a case for governments, international organizations and other stakeholders (WHO 2008).

More specifically, the Dementia India Report, released on World Alzheimer's Day 2010, clearly defines the social and economic impact of the condition, highlighting eight recommendations (see Box 10.2) that need to be considered. The document calls upon the government to recognize dementia as a public and social welfare priority and develop a national dementia strategy. The integration of dementia care services through the primary health care system, with the possible use of non-specialist health care workers, is a likely answer to the public health concern in this part of the region.

Box 10.2 Key messages for policy makers (recommendations of the Dementia India Report)

1. Make dementia a national priority.
2. Increase funding for dementia research.
3. Increase awareness about dementia.
4. Improve dementia identification and skills for care.
5. Develop community support.
6. Guarantee caregiver support packages.
7. Develop comprehensive dementia care models.
8. Develop new national policies and legislation for people with dementia.

Conclusion

Both at the state and at the central level, government in India has started to respond to the cause. Efforts are on to include services for people with dementia as one of the items in the next five-year plan for the country, the revised national mental health programme, and the national policy for older people. The country is in a much better position than it was a decade ago, as far as services for people with dementia are concerned. However, a lot more needs to be done to bridge the treatment gap. We have progressed considerably from research to a position where we can produce evidence-based interventions to influence health policy. We are optimistic that the next few years will see a lot more change in this direction. Now is the time for action!

References

10/66 Dementia Research Group (2004) 'Care arrangements for people with dementia in developing countries.' *International Journal of Geriatric Psychiatry 19*, 2, 170–177.

Alzheimer's and Related Disorders Society of India (2010) *The Dementia India Report: Prevalence, Impact, Costs and Services for Dementia.* New Delhi: Alzheimer's and Related Disorders Society of India.

Alzheimer's Disease International (2006) *Dementia in the Asian Pacific Region: The Epidemic is Here.* Available at www.alz.co.uk/research/files/apreport.pdf

Cummings, J.L., Mega, M., Gray, K., Rosenberg-Thompson, S. *et al.* (1994) 'The Neuropsychiatric Inventory: comprehensive assessment of psychopathology in dementia.' *Neurology 44*, 12, 2308–2314.

Dias, A. and Patel, V. (2009) 'Closing the treatment gap for dementia in India.' *Indian Journal of Psychiatry 51*, 5, 93–97.

Dias, A., Dewey, M.E., D'Souza, J., Dhume, R. *et al.* (2008) 'The effectiveness of a home care program for supporting caregivers of persons with dementia in developing countries: A randomized controlled trial from Goa, India.' *PLoS ONE 3*, 6, e2333.

Dias, A., Samuel, R., Patel, V., Prince, M., Parameshwaran, R. and Krishnamoorthy, E.S. (2004) 'The impact associated with caring for a person with dementia: a report from the 10/66 Dementia Research Group's Indian network.' *International Journal of Geriatric Psychiatry 19*, 2, 182–184.

Ferri, C.P., Ames, D. and Prince, M. (2004) 'Behavioral and psychological symptoms of dementia in developing countries.' *International Psychogeriatrics 16*, 441–459.

Fillenbaum, G., Chandra, V. and Ganguli, M. (1999) 'Development of an activities of daily living scale to screen for dementia in an illiterate rural older population in India.' *Age and Ageing 28*, 2, 161–168.

NISD (National Institute of Social Defense, Ministry of Social Justice and Empowerment, Government of India) (2008) *Age Care in India: National Initiative on Care for Elderly.*

Patel, V. and Prince, M. (2001) 'Ageing and mental health in a developing country: who cares? Qualitative studies from Goa, India.' *Psychological Medicine 31*, 1, 29–38.

Prince, M.J., Acosta, D., Castro-Costa, E., Jackson, J. and Shaji, K.S. (2009) 'Packages of care for dementia in low- and middle-income countries.' *PLoS.Med 6*, 11, e1000176.

Saxena, S., Thornicroft, G., Knapp, M. and Whiteford, H. (2007) 'Resources for mental health: scarcity, inequity, and inefficiency.' *Lancet 370*, 9590, 878–889.

Shaji, K.S., Kishore, A.N.R., Lal, K.P. and Prince, M. (2002) 'Revealing a hidden problem: an evaluation of a community dementia case-finding program from the Indian 10/66 dementia research network.' *International Journal of Geriatric Psychiatry 17*, 222–225. doi:10.1002/gps.553

World Health Organization, Department of Health Promotion (2002) 'Health and aging: a discussion paper.' Presented at the Second United Nations Assembly on Aging in Madrid. Geneva: World Health Organization.

World Health Organization. mhGAP (2008) 'Mental Health Gap Action Program. Scaling up care for mental, neurological and substance use disorders: programs and plans.' Geneva: World Health Organization.

Zarit, S.H., Reeve, K.E. and Bach-Peterson, J. (1980) 'Relatives of the impaired elderly: correlates of feelings of burden.' *The Gerontologist 20*, 6, 649–655.

Chapter 11

Evaluating the Impact of Environmental Design on Physical Activity Levels of Individuals Living with a Dementia in Residential Accommodation

Loren deVries and Victoria Traynor

Introduction

The beneficial effects of physical activity on health care outcomes for aging populations, and more specifically for individuals living with a dementia, have been well established by international researchers across a range of disciplines and care settings. The benefits for individuals living with a dementia included improved daily functioning, sleep and mood, and decreased fears, disorientation, agitated pacing and restless circuiting (Weuve *et al.* 2004; Zeisel 2006). Environmental design in residential accommodation was also recognised as an important therapeutic source to promote the well-being of older people, in particular individuals living with a dementia (Marshall 1998; Powell *et al.* 2000). Environmental design enhanced cognitive and physical capacities of individuals living with a dementia (Parker *et al.* 2004). It is therefore hypothesised that promoting physical activity levels among individuals living with a dementia in residential accommodation will improve their health care outcomes.

Since there is strong evidence about the positive impact of physical activity on health care outcomes of populations across the age span, and the influence of the environment in determining physical activity levels, it is useful to explore the effect of environmental design of residential accommodation on physical activity levels among individuals living with a dementia. Only recently, empirical evidence became available on this very issue, with specific reference to individuals living with a dementia (King 2001). The aim of this chapter is to report findings from a research project which demonstrated how environmental design contributed to low physical activity levels among individuals living with a dementia in residential accommodation. Recommendations are made for practitioners, education providers, managers and policy makers on how to make small-scale amendments to existing environmental designs in residential accommodation to promote physical activity among individuals living with a dementia and contribute to improvements in their health care outcomes.

Project aims and objectives

The aim was to:

- identify how environmental design in residential accommodation (i) promoted and (ii) inhibited physical activity levels among individuals living with a dementia.

The specific objectives were to:

- measure physical activity levels (duration, type and location) among individuals living with a dementia in residential accommodation (observation charts and accelerometers)

- record footwear type (observation charts)

- evaluate environmental design features of residential accommodation for individuals living with a dementia (observation charts, audits and photographs)

- identify what staff consider are important features of environmental design in residential accommodation for promoting physical activity levels among individuals living with a dementia (focus groups).

The focus of this chapter is the findings from (i) observation charts used to measure physical activity levels of individuals living with a dementia and (ii) audits to evaluate the environmental design of residential accommodation. Other findings are reported elsewhere (deVries, Traynor and Humpel 2010; Traynor and deVries 2009; Traynor, deVries and Humpel 2009).

Influencing clinical practice and enhancing the lives of individuals living with a dementia

This chapter is for you if you are a practitioner, manager, education provider or policy maker with responsibilities to provide care for individuals living with a dementia in residential accommodation. We know that each of you can influence the environmental design of residential accommodation for individuals living with a dementia. We intend this chapter to provide you with the motivation and recommendations to make amendments to environmental design which increase physical activity levels and contribute to improved health care outcomes for individuals living with a dementia. To set the scene, we have created Case study 11.1 from positive examples of environmental design and physical activity from the findings of this project. Please take time to read this case study and consider the questions listed at the end of it.

CASE STUDY 11.1 HOW ENVIRONMENTAL DESIGN PROMOTED PHYSICAL ACTIVITY FOR DULCIE

I'm Dulcie. I waken and decide to get up. I swing my legs easily out of my bed and into my slippers. I smell something pleasant and hear a gentle hustle and bustle. I'll head toward them. I lean out of my door and see daylight beaming at the end of my hallway. My legs won't move easily, but it's not far, so I give it a go... After my meal, I easily find a comfy armchair to sit in... A friendly face asks if I'd like to join others for tea and scones on the veranda. I go outside and feel the warm sun on my body. I enjoy watching some children playing... A nice man asks if I want to join a game of indoor bowls. I've never liked it. He asks if I'd rather go for a walk and pick some herbs. That's a good idea. It looks like a long way, but I see a bench... I see people laughing through the window. I'll head inside. The path loops around so it's easy to find the door. I'm out of puff but there are lots of chairs to choose from, so I sit and watch the end of the game... I hear cups and saucers clinking. I feel tired and can't be bothered. I'll ask them to bring me my tea, but the nurse tells me Mary is waiting. That sounds nice but my legs won't go. The nurse gives me an arm and a little encouragement – I'm off. It's not as far as I thought and I enjoy my cuppa with Mary... I want to walk back to my room but feel unsure of the way. I look around and see a familiar green colour. I head towards the green and find a familiar photograph on a door. I enjoy a break standing at a window watching the comings and goings... A nurse asks me where I'd like my dinner. Sitting here on my chair sounds best. The nurse tries to encourage me to join my friends, but I want to stay here in the quiet. She brings my dinner and I enjoy it... Getting ready for bed. What a nice feeling inside. Must've been a good day...

Answer these questions:

- List the ways in which the environmental design promoted physical activity for Dulcie.

- Compare where Dulcie lives with the residential accommodation where you work.

- Compare the opportunities Dulcie had to engage in physical activity with those in the residential accommodation where you work.

- How is the well-being of Dulcie promoted? Compare this with the residential accommodation where you work.

This activity will enable you to make best use of the content and the research findings presented. Completing this activity will enable you to more carefully and meaningfully consider the implications of the findings presented in this chapter. It is intended that these questions will trigger your interest in furthering your knowledge and understanding about this chapter.

Background

In 2009 there were an estimated 245,500 individuals living with a dementia in Australia with an almost fivefold rise of 1.3 million individuals projected by 2050 (Access Economics 2009a). These prevalence rates are similar to those in other developed nations. Up to 40 per cent of individuals with a diagnosis of dementia (just under 100,000) in Australia are living in residential accommodation (Access Economics 2009b). Dementia is a National Health Priority in Australia with an integrated funding model for dementia clinical teams, education and research (Department of Health and Ageing 2006). The project reported here is a collaboration with the NSW/ACT Dementia Training Study Centre, the University of Wollongong and Warrigal Care. The focus of the project was the impact of environmental design in residential accommodation on physical activity levels of individuals living with dementia.

PHYSICAL ACTIVITY

Physical activity was defined as (i) incidental activities of daily living and (ii) physical training (Leone, Deudon and Robert 2008). Promotion of increased physical activity levels among older people is important because it decreases the risk of injury, improves health-related quality of life, enhances psychological status and improves mobility and physical functioning (Mulrow *et al.* 1994; Sallis *et al.* 1997; Williams *et al.* 2005). The ability to perform everyday activities independently can deteriorate with age when age-associated chronic diseases are experienced. Independence and the ability to live in the community are compromised when there is a loss or deterioration in mobility, muscle strength, balance and mental health (Netz, Axelrad and Argov 2007). Deteriorations of these capabilities were commonly found to be due to reduced physical activity levels (Dobbs *et al.* 2005). Older people have a great need to maintain physical activity levels as this has an impact on their overall quality of life and independent functioning (Bassey 1997).

Individuals living with a dementia in residential accommodation were found to be less physically active because of the social stigma associated with dementia, environmental barriers and attitudes of health care providers (Williams *et al.* 2005). Personal characteristics and the inability to initiate activity also contributed to decreased physical activity levels (Warms, Belza and Whitney 2007). Individuals living with a dementia benefited from increased physical activity levels, with decreased behavioural problems, such as agitated wandering and aggression (Algase *et al.* 1997; Torrington 2007; Woodhead *et al.* 2005). Other benefits were improved quality of life, decreased falls, reduced incidence of constipation and decreased use of restraints (Brawley 2001; Paw *et al.* 2008).

Opportunities for activity, such as places to walk, are important for older people (Lawton 2001). Within residential accommodation, safety issues often restrict opportunities to move around and make the most of the environment in a facility, in particular for those with a dementia (Fleming, Crookes and Sum 2008). Staff may restrict movement because of their fear that a fall might be sustained by the older residents for whom they are caring (Morgan and Stewart 1999). Inactivity and lack of sensory stimulation are described as the enemies of quality of life (Lawton 2001), and increased well-being is associated with increased activity levels (Parker *et al.* 2004). Research with community-dwelling populations demonstrated a link between environments and physical activity levels: the environment determined physical activity levels (duration and type), and changed environments improved physical activity levels (Sallis *et al.* 1997). The benefits of increasing physical activity levels for older people have been clearly documented, but there remains a gap about the impact of environmental design on physical activity levels among those living in residential accommodation.

ENVIRONMENT

A recent literature review demonstrated that specific environmental design features promoted a more positive experience of dementia (Fleming, Crookes and Sum 2008). Environmental design is a major contributor to human behaviour, quality of life and quality of care (Torrington *et al.* 2004). Homelike environments, such as personalised rooms with domestic furnishings, are associated with enhanced interaction, reduced agitation and improved well-being (Calkins 2001; Gitlin, Liebman and Winter 2003). Personalised belongings promote positive behaviours and assist in maintaining personal identities (Sloane *et al.* 1998). It is not uncommon in some residential accommodation facilities to see individuals living with a dementia experiencing agitated wandering, calling out and talking anxiously to themselves. This is prevented with specific environmental designs in residential accommodation.

In Australia, 40 per cent of individuals living with a dementia move from their own homes into residential accommodation (Access Economics 2009b). This high incidence rate demonstrates the importance of attending to environmental designs to promote positive living for individuals with a dementia in residential accommodation. The design of residential accommodation should reflect what we know about the structure and activity of the brain and socio-psychological needs of individuals living with a dementia (Zeisel 2006). The environment should assist individuals living with a dementia to function more independently by enhancing memories and promoting functioning in parts of the brain which continue to do well. Recommendations for the design of residential accommodation specifically for individuals living with a dementia were available as long ago as 1998 (Marshall 1998). Design guides offer architects and managers recommendations on how to build residential accommodation to promote the well-being of individuals living with a dementia (Day, Carreon and Stump 2000). One way to promote the use of these guides is to provide practitioners, education providers, managers and policy makers with feedback about the impact of their environmental design on individuals living with a dementia within their residential accommodation.

There are a range of ways to measure the environmental design of residential accommodation, including that designed specifically for individuals living with a dementia (Cunningham 2008; Cutler *et al.* 2006; Fleming, Forbes and Bennett 2003; Powell *et al.* 2000; Slaughter *et al.* 2006; Sloane *et al.* 2002; Torrington *et al.* 2008):

- Environmental Audit Tool (EAT)

- Design for Dementia: Audit Tool (DDAT)

- Evaluation of Older People's Living Environments (EVOLVE)
- Professional Environmental Assessment Protocol (PEAP)
- Sheffield Care Environment Assessment Matrix (SCEAM)
- Therapeutic Environment Screening Survey for Nursing Homes (TESS-NH).

The SCEAM evaluates (i) environmental design (building design) and (ii) how the care environment (building use) is used by residents and staff (Torrington 2007; Torrington *et al.* 2004). The SCEAM, recommended for use to develop models of care and in research projects (Parker *et al.* 2004), provided evidence of correlations between building design and quality of life for residents living in the building being evaluated. The SCEAM items were developed from research with architects and advanced practitioners working with older people (Torrington 2007; Torrington *et al.* 2004). The SCEAM was valid, reliable, contemporary, simple to use and required a short turnaround for data entry and analysis.

Method

This was a mixed method project in which qualitative and quantitative data collection and analysis techniques were adopted (Creswell and Plano-Clark 2010). The project was undertaken by researchers in the disciplines of nursing, physiotherapy and psychology. A dissemination strategy included a one-day workshop at the end of the project in which clinical teams developed action plans for making amendments to environmental designs to increase physical activity levels of individuals living with a dementia in the residential accommodation where they worked. The project was an example of an implementation project in which knowledge translation has been achieved by the research team (Rycroft-Malone 2004).

ETHICS AND RECRUITMENT

This project was approved by the Human Research Ethics Committee (HREC) at the University of Wollongong, and the Chief Executive Officer (CEO) of Warrigal Care provided permission to seek participation from six nominated residential accommodation facilities. Initial agreement for the project to be undertaken at these six residential accommodation facilities was sought from the managers. Information sessions about the project were held to seek permission from staff, residents and visitors to undertake the project. Posters were placed on noticeboards at facilities to promote awareness about the project. Information sessions and posters emphasised that if any staff member, resident or visitor did not want to be included in the project, specifically the observation data, they were invited to contact someone from the research team or a member of staff to inform us or them of this. No member of staff, resident or visitor made a request not to be included within the project.

SAMPLE AND SETTING

The partner organisation, Warrigal Care, was a not-for-profit aged care provider of 'aging in place' accommodation for older people: independent living, hostel accommodation and nursing homes. They provided services across the Illawarra, NSW, Australia, which was categorised as a regional area. The six residential accommodation facilities provided included dementia-specific services. The individual participants consisted of staff, residents and visitors who worked at, lived in and visited the six nominated facilities. The residents who participated consisted of a wide range of older people. In regards to dementia, there were individuals living with (i) a formal medical diagnosis of dementia; (ii) cognitive impairment which was not formally diagnosed; and (iii) no cognitive impairment. Exclusively collecting data about individuals living with a dementia requires staff resources from the participating facility to record data, but this was not available for this project.

DATA COLLECTION

A range of qualitative and quantitative data were generated (Cramer 2003; Creswell and Plano-Clark 2010; Silverman 2005) during this project. The quantitative physical activity observation and environmental audits are reported here.

PHYSICAL ACTIVITY OBSERVATIONS

The observations were recorded in nominated target areas of each facility. Target areas were identified following a review of floor plans and visits to facilities, and varied according to the size and usual activities undertaken within a facility. Target areas consisted of communal areas, such as dining rooms and outside areas. No private areas, such as bedrooms and bathrooms of the residents, were included in the observations. Managers described the usual routines of the facilities, and the following schedule of observations was developed:

- Observations 1 (O1): two hours' post-commencement of day shift activities.

- Observations 2 (O2): 30 minutes' pre-lunchtime activities.

- Observations 3 (O3): one hour's post-dinnertime activities.

An observation chart was created to record the duration, type and location of physical activity by the older people living in the residential accommodation. The charts were completed by hand, using pen and paper. Stopwatches were used to time the duration, in seconds, of resident movements. Residents often participated in several physical activity events in each time period and were allocated their own stopwatch to ensure accuracy of recording observations. The type of movement was recorded onto the observation charts using a coded entry. The data were entered into an Excel spreadsheet.

Environmental audit

Each facility was assessed using direct observation and the SCEAM checklist of desired building features, which were shown to be beneficial for individuals living with a dementia. SCEAM created 300 individual coded features in ten domains. Each feature was scored as 'present' or 'absent', and each domain had the potential to reach a total score of 100 per cent. The SCEAM results were represented as ten different percentages, one for each of the ten domains. Each facility had two sets of percentages: (i) building design and (ii) building use. A final score (expressed as a percentage) was created after the scoring and used to make comparisons between (i) environments and (ii) domains.

Data analysis

Data analysis consisted of descriptive statistical analysis (Creswell and Plano-Clark 2010). Means and standard deviations were created for the physical activity events observed and the SCEAM domains within building design and building use. Means and standard deviations were created for each facility and across the six participating facilities. The findings are presented in bar charts (Figures 11.1–11.5) to highlight the importance of the findings.

Findings

The focus of the findings in this chapter is the physical activity observations and environmental audits.

Sites and participants

The care was provided by the six residential accommodation facilities (Facilities 1, 2, 3, 4, 5 and 6). The care provided consisted of:

- 'low care' (hostel-type accommodation) (n=2)
- 'high care' (nursing-home-type accommodation) (n=4).

The population within the residential accommodation facilities ranged from 60 to 100 older people. Most residential accommodation facilities were purpose-built for older people (n=5). Three of the facilities were not new builds and had within them a range of environmental design flaws for individuals living with a dementia. Four of the facilities provided dementia-specific services (Facilities 1, 2, 4 and 5) and the other two (Facilities 3 and 6) provided care for individuals living with a dementia but without specialist services, such as specifically experienced staff.

The number and range of older people undertaking physical activity events reflected the size of the residential accommodation in which they lived. During the project, a total of 913 older people were observed undertaking physical activity events across the six participating facilities (Figure 11.1).

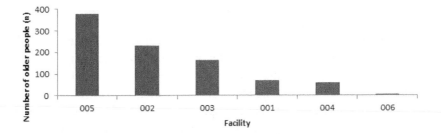

Figure 11.1 Summary of the number of older people (n) undertaking physical activity events by facility

A total of 76 per cent of the physical activity events were undertaken by older women and 10 per cent were undertaken by older people from culturally and linguistically diverse communities.

PHYSICAL ACTIVITY
Physical activity levels among older people living within the six participating residential accommodation facilities were observed as follows:

- 3 × 7-hour observation periods × 3 different days (up to 21 hours per facility), with a total of 110 hours' observation.

A total of 1540 physical activity events were recorded, with a mean number of 257 physical activity events (sd ±272) across the six facilities. The wide variability in these data was due to the different sizes of the residential accommodation facilities. What is more meaningful to look at is the mean number of physical activity events per resident, which ranged from only

1 to 3 (sd ±1) (Figure 11.2). Facility 2 had the highest physical activity levels: up to three times more than at the other five facilities.

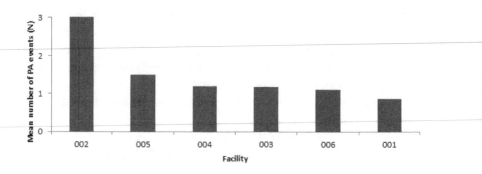

Figure 11.2 Summary of mean physical activity (PA) events for each resident by facility

The mean length of time spent undertaking physical activity events across all facilities was two minutes (sd ±1 minute). We found that just under 5 per cent of all physical activity events were undertaken with staff members in the residential accommodation. The physical activity events mostly took place in only a few of the target areas. For example, just under half of all the physical activity events (44%) took place in the dining areas over the three days of observation of each facility. The next most common areas for recording of physical activity events were the craft and outdoor areas. The time of day was also important, with most physical activity events occurring at lunchtime or after evening meals. The weekends increased physical activity events undertaken by residents when visitors came and the residents walked in the outdoor areas, but the number of physical activity events never increased above three events.

ENVIRONMENTAL AUDIT

The SCEAM scores for the domain of 'staff' across building design and building use were the highest scores at all facilities, reaching 95 per cent (sd ± 7 per cent) for both aspects of the environmental design. This demonstrates that practitioners were making attempts to use their environment positively. The mean score for the domain of 'physical' (accessibility of entrances and within rooms, handrails, lighting and obstacles) was 65 per cent (sd ± 15 per cent) for building design and building use (Figure 11.3).

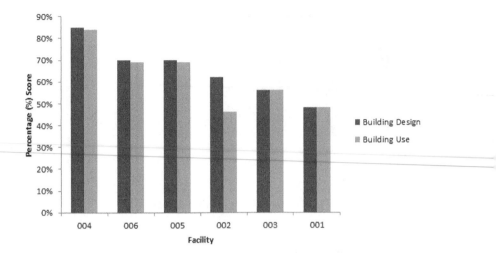

Figure 11.3 SCEAM percentage (%) score for 'physical' by building design and building use and facility

Facility 4, which had the highest score, was a brand new building and had opened only weeks prior to the project commencing. Facility 2, which had the lowest score, had obstacles in many of the target areas which were observed. Photographs of both these facilities provided useful data to complement the environmental audits to demonstrate qualitative aspects within building design and building use.

All the facilities scored low in the area of 'cognitive' building design and building use (internal landmarks; colour-coded loop routes to mobilise; way-finding signals), with mean scores of 38 and 37 per cent respectively (sd ± 8 per cent) (Figure 11.4).

Only one third of the building design in the facilities was considered to be sensitive to the cognitive needs of individuals living with a dementia. The four facilities which provided dementia-specific services (Facilities 1, 2, 4 and 5) did not score best in this category. Facility 3 does not have dementia-specific services, but this facility scored highest for cognitive building design and use for individuals living with a dementia.

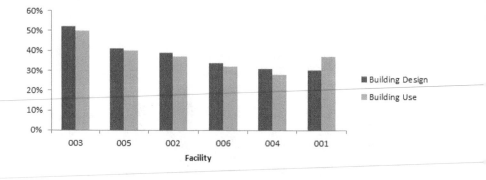

*Figure 11.4 SCEAM percentage (%) score for 'cognition' by
building design and building use and facility*

The greatest variability was recorded within the domain of 'personalisation'
(personalised spaces and photos; varying chairs; and shelves for personal
items), both between facilities and within the building design and use aspects
of the domains (Figure 11.5).

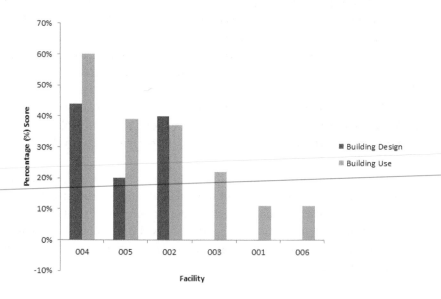

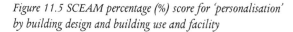

*Figure 11.5 SCEAM percentage (%) score for 'personalisation'
by building design and building use and facility*

In the domain of 'personalisation', building use scores were higher than
building design scores, with means of 30 and 17 per cent respectively.
Thus, staff used the building in a more personalised way than its original

building design suggested. Even within the brand-new Facility 4, the score was low in the domain of personalisation within building design. Facilities 1, 3 and 6 scored 0 per cent for their building design within the domain of personalisation.

Discussion

The findings demonstrated that the physical activity levels of individuals living with a dementia in the residential accommodation were influenced by the environmental design of the facility. Overall physical activity levels were poor, which replicated the findings of other researchers (Voelkl *et al.* 2003). Despite well-documented evidence about the benefits of physical activity, we found that older people living in residential accommodation were not regularly participating in physical activity of a meaningfully sustained duration. Physical activity that was observed was incidental and occurred mainly when the residents walked to have meals in the dining area or used bathroom facilities. Minimal physical activity occurred in outdoor areas, meaning that residents are spending most of their time indoors. Exits to outside areas required navigation to locate, and at times the doors were locked or closed. Outdoor areas that are easier to find and ensure a transition from inside to outside may assist residents to spend more time outside. We found that the older people living in the residential accommodation were motivated to move from one area of the facility to another when there were activities which attracted their interest. The research team was one of these attractions. We found that our presence drew many older people from their usual places to come and talk with the team about the research.

- The high SCEAM scores within the 'staff' domain demonstrated that staff were provided with an environment that meets their needs, but other scores demonstrated that the environmental design did not meet the basic needs of the residents.

- The scores demonstrated that the domain of 'physical aspects' of the environment was reasonable. Staff were able to adjust building use and make amendments for individuals living with a dementia, which overcame negative aspects in the building design.

- The 'cognitive' scores demonstrated that the environmental design was potentially toxic to individuals living with a dementia. Within this domain, staff showed that they had not overcome the building design flaws, because the building use score was equally low.

- The most stark SCEAM score finding was found within the domain of 'personalisation'. Some of the facilities had a zero score for building design, demonstrating a lack of attempt to attend to this domain by architects designing and managers commissioning the building of residential accommodation for older people. A hospital-like, rather than a home-like, building design prevailed in all the facilities. The higher score within building use in the domain of personalisation demonstrates how staff made active attempts to overcome these flaws in building design, but it was clear that it would be extremely difficult to overcome a score of zero, even with creative approaches to building use.

As long ago as 1998, Marshall explained that poor environmental design was disabling for individuals living with a dementia. The findings from this project demonstrate that we have not developed our learning sufficiently to amend building design or building use to promote the cognitive capacities of individuals living with a dementia.

These data would be usefully fed back to policy makers when considering the regulation of buildings for residential accommodation. Perhaps consumer input could also be used to persuade a move away from non-personalised building design towards a more personalised and home-like environment, to promote a more positive experience for individuals living with a dementia. A more home-like environment would enable individuals living with a dementia to engage more easily with their environment, explore, and undertake incidental physical activity.

Strengths and limitations

This project adopted a mixed method research design, and a wide range of data was generated to explain the impact of environmental design on physical activity levels of individuals with a dementia living in residential accommodation. The large number of observations of physical activity events provided an in-depth description of the duration, location and type of physical activity levels among individuals with a dementia living in residential accommodation. This is one of several studies which have provided data in this area of dementia care. The SCEAM provided environmental audits across ten domains of building design and an understanding about the positive and negative aspects of environmental design in the participating residential accommodation facilities. The project concluded with an action-planning workshop for all six participating facilities. Staff members drew on the findings from the project to develop a project plan for making amendments to environmental design in the residential accommodation where they worked, including outcomes for measuring achievements in increasing physical activity levels among individuals living with a dementia.

The facilities included those which provided dementia-specific services as well as those which were more general aged-care residential accommodation. In future projects it would be worthwhile considering an observation study limited to dementia-specific units, to build on the data generated from this project. The data entry of the environmental audits was time-consuming, and a computer-generated package on a device such as an iPad would increase the efficiency of data collection. Recruiting and mentoring staff members to collect the data from the residential accommodation facility in which they work would increase the likelihood that the findings would be implemented at the end of the research project (Rycroft-Malone 2004).

RECOMMENDATIONS FOR PRACTICE

Evidence was well established about the benefits of physical activity for older people, particularly for individuals living with a dementia, but in practice it was found that there were unacceptably low physical activity levels among older people living in residential accommodation. In the main, the only observable physical activity was incidental and consisted of ambulation to have a meal in a dining area or to use bathroom facilities. The recommendations from this project focus on how environmental design amendments can be used to promote physical activity levels among older people, particularly those living with a dementia. The recommendations from this project focus on how environmental design can be used specifically to promote an increase in incidental physical activity levels (Box 11.1).

Box 11.1 Summary recommendations for amendments to environmental design to increase physical activity in residential accommodation for individuals living with a dementia

---

Recommended amendments to environmental design:

- longer distance between dining area and rooms with resting places along the way
- corridors with no dead ends
- handrails in appropriate places
- way-finding cues
- personalised entry doors
- adequate lighting

- comfortable temperature
- easily accessible outdoor areas
- outdoor areas with a view
- home-like environment
- staff-aided walking.

The environmental design amendments suggested are achievable in most residential accommodation facilities, as demonstrated by those participating residential accommodation facilities which scored higher on the building use aspect of the domains compared to the building design score. The findings demonstrated that practitioners and managers use creative approaches to overcome obstacles caused by environmental design.

Conclusion

This project clearly shows that the mean of one physical activity event (lasting on average two minutes) unequivocally demonstrates low physical activity levels among individuals living with a dementia in residential accommodation. Aspects of environmental design in the residential accommodation which influenced physical activity levels among individuals living with dementia were demonstrated by the low SCEAM scores in the domains of building design and use for 'cognition' and building design for 'personalisation'. The SCEAM scores were higher within building use in the domain of personalisation. This demonstrated that staff and managers created an environment which increased physical activity levels among those without a dementia, but the amendments were not sufficiently sensitive to promote physical activity levels among those individuals living with a dementia in residential accommodation, or among older people.

These findings can be used by practitioners, managers, education providers and policy makers to make environmental action plans for the residential accommodation where they are responsible for providing services to individuals living with dementia.

A more recent project undertaken by this research team found that a men's exercise programme, including the role of a male exercise scientist, had a positive impact on the experience of dementia and the physical capacities of the participants (Traynor *et al.* 2010). Future research will include a partnership with a not-for-profit university gym service and a group of individuals with younger onset dementia living in residential accommodation, and a larger-scale physical activity intervention study.

Another testimony to the importance of the environment came in 1997 from a person living with dementia herself:

> I don't want to be
> inside
> Anywhere at all
> It's much too hot and
> bright
> It just don't feel right
> at all
> I need fresh air –
> I keep calling out
> 'Nurse, nurse, carry
> me to where I were
> lying on grass'

(Killick 1997, p.39)

This poem was created from words spoken by a person with dementia when she was talking with John Killick, who was a 'writer in residence' for the Stirling Dementia Services Development Centre (Killick 1997).

Returning now to the case study of Dulcie (see page 206): the environment in which Dulcie lived promoted opportunities for her to feel her outside environment and participate in incidental physical activity as well as physical training. Dulcie was able to experience the benefits of physical activity in her daily life, and for her the experience of living with a dementia was more positive than it was for the person speaking in the poem above.

Think about the key findings from this project and how practitioners, education providers, managers and policy makers use the environment in ways that either promote or inhibit physical activity levels among individuals living with a dementia in residential accommodation. We conclude by asking you to reflect on what amendments you can make to the environmental design where you work, so as to enable individuals living with a dementia, like to the woman speaking in the poem above, to experience the positive benefits of health care outcomes associated with physical activity in their daily lives.

References

Access Economics (2009a) *Keeping Dementia Front of Mind: Incidence and Prevalence 2009–2050.* Canberra: Alzheimer's Australia.

Access Economics (2009b) *Making Choices. Future Dementia Care: Projections, Problems and Preferences.* Canberra: Alzheimer's Australia.

Algase, D.L., Kupferschmid, B., Beel-Bates, C.A. and Beattie, E.R. (1997) 'Estimates of stability of daily wandering behaviour among cognitively impaired long-term care residents.' *Nursing 46,* 3, 172–178.

Bassey, E.J. (1997) 'Physical capabilities, exercise and aging.' *Reviews in Clinical Gerontology 7,* 289–297.

Brawley, E.C. (2001) 'Environmental design for Alzheimer's disease: a quality of life issue.' *Aging and Mental Health 5*, 1, S79–S83.

Calkins, M.P. (2001) 'The physical and social environment of the person with Alzheimer's disease.' *Aging and Mental Health 5*, 1, S74–S78.

Cramer, D. (2003) *Advanced Quantitative Data Analysis.* Philadelphia, PA: Open University Press.

Creswell, J.W. and Plano-Clark, V. (2010) *Designing and Conducting Mixed Methods Research.* London: Sage.

Cunningham, C. (2008) *Design for People with Dementia: Audit Tool.* Stirling: Dementia Services Development Centre.

Cutler, L.J., Kane, R.A., Degenholtz, H.B., Miller, M.J. and Grant, L. (2006) 'Assessing and comparing physical environments for nursing home residents: using new tools for greater research specificity.' *The Gerontologist 46*, 1, 42–51.

Day, K., Carreon, D. and Stump, C. (2000) 'The therapeutic design of environments for people with dementia: a review of the empirical research.' *The Gerontologist 40*, 4, 397–416.

Department of Health and Ageing (2006) *Dementia: A National Health Priority.* Canberra: Department of Health and Ageing.

deVries, L., Traynor, V. and Humpel, N. (2010) 'Evaluating the impact of the environment on physical activity levels for individuals living with a dementia in residential aged care facilities.' Poster presentation for Stirling Dementia Services Development Centre Annual Conference in London, October 2010.

Dobbs, D., Munn, J., Zimmerman, S., Boustani, M. *et al.* (2005) 'Characteristics associated with lower activity involvement in long-term residents with dementia.' *The Gerontologist 45*, 1, 81–86.

Fleming, R., Crookes, P. and Sum, S. (2008) 'Review of the role of technology and environmental design in delivering better care outcomes for people with dementia.' Unpublished report. Dementia Collaborative Research Centre, University of New South Wales, Sydney.

Fleming, R., Forbes, I. and Bennett, K. (2003) *Adapting the Ward for People with Dementia.* Sydney: NSW Department of Health.

Gitlin, L.N., Liebman, J. and Winter, L. (2003) 'Are environmental interventions effective in the management of Alzheimer's disease and related disorders?' *Alzheimer's Care Quarterly 4*, 2, 85–107.

Killick, J. (1997) *You are Words.* (Dementia poems.) London: Hawker.

King, A.C. (2001) 'Interventions to promote physical activity by older adults.' *Journals of Gerontology, 56A*, 36–46.

Lawton, M.P. (2001) 'The physical environment of the person with Alzheimer's disease.' *Aging and Mental Health 5* (S1), S-64.

Leone, E., Deudon, A. and Robert, P. (2008) 'Physical activity, dementia and BPSD.' *Journal of Nutrition, Health and Aging 12*, 7, 457–462.

Marshall, M. (1998) 'Therapeutic Buildings for People with Dementia.' In S. Judd, M. Marshall and P. Phippen (eds) *Design in Dementia.* London: *Journal of Dementia Care.*

Morgan, D.G. and Stewart, N.J. (1999) 'The physical environment of special care units: needs of residents with dementia from the perspective of staff and family caregivers.' *Qualitative Health Research 9*, 1, 105–118.

Mulrow, C.D., Gerety, M.B., Kanten, D., Cornell, J.E. *et al.* (1994) 'A randomized trial of physical rehabilitation for very frail nursing home residents.' *American Medical Association 271*, 7, 519–524.

Netz, Y., Axelrad, S. and Argov, E. (2007) 'Group physical activity for demented older adults – feasibility and effectiveness.' *Clinical Rehabilitation 21*, 977–986.

Parker, C., Barnes, S., McKee, K., Morgan, K., Torrington, J. and Tregenza, P. (2004) 'Quality of life and building design in residential and nursing homes for older people.' *Ageing and Society 24*, 941–962.

Paw, C.A., van Uffelen, M.J., Riphagen, I. and van Mechelen, W. (2008) 'The functional effects of physical exercise training in frail older people: a systematic review.' *Sports Medicine 38*, 9, 781–793.

Powell, M.P., Weisman, G.D., Sloane, P., Norris-Baker, C., Calkins, M. and Zimmerman, S.I. (2000) 'Professional Environmental Assessment Procedure for special care units for elders with dementing illness and its relationship to the therapeutic environment screening schedule.' *Alzheimer's Disease and Associated Disorders 14*, 1, 28–38.

Rycroft-Malone, J. (2004) 'The PARIHS framework: a framework for guiding the implementation of evidence-based practice.' *Journal of Nursing Care Quality 19*, 4, 297–304.

Sallis, J.F., Johnson, M.F., Calfas, K.J., Caparosa, S. and Nichols, J.F. (1997) 'Assessing the perceived physical environmental variables that may influence physical activity.' *Physical Education, Recreation and Dance* 68, 4, 345–351.

Silverman, D. (2005) *Doing Qualitative Research: A Practical Handbook,* 2nd edition. London: Sage.

Slaughter, S., Calkins, M., Eliasziw, M. and Reimer, M. (2006) 'Measuring physical and social environments in nursing homes for people with middle to late stage dementia.' *Journal of the American Geriatrics Society* 54, 9, 1436–1441.

Sloane, P.D., Mitchell, C.M., Preisser, J.S., Phillips, C. *et al.* (1998) 'Environmental correlates of resident agitation in Alzheimer's disease special care units.' *Journal of the American Geriatrics Society* 46, 7, 862–869.

Sloane, P.D., Mitchell, C.M., Weisman, G., Zimmerman, S. *et al.* (2002) 'The Therapeutic Environment Screening Survey for Nursing Homes (TESS-NH): an observational instrument for assessing the physical environment of institutional settings for persons with dementia.' *The Journals of Gerontology* 57B, 2, S69–S78.

Torrington, J. (2007) 'Evaluating quality of life in residential care buildings.' *Building Research and Information* 35, 5, 514–528.

Torrington, J., Barnes, S., McKee, K., Morgan, K. and Tregenza, P. (2004) 'The influence of building design on the quality of life of older people.' *Architectural Science Review* 47, 2, 193–197.

Torrington, J., Barnes, S., McKee, K. *et al.* (2008) *Evaluation of Older People's Living Environment (EVOLVE).* Sheffield: University of Sheffield.

Traynor, V. and deVries, L. (2009) 'Evaluating the impact of the environment on physical activity levels for individuals living with a dementia in residential aged care facilities.' Oral presentation at Australian Association of Gerontology, NSW Annual Rural Conference, Broken Hill, April 2009.

Traynor, V., deVries, L. and Humpel, N. (2009) 'Evaluating the impact of the environment on physical activity levels for individuals living with a dementia in residential aged care facilities.' Unpublished report, University of Wollongong, Wollongong.

Traynor, V., Olbrecht, T., Smith, E. and Woods, J. (2010) 'Using the environment: evaluating a physical activity programme for older men living with dementia in residential aged care facilities.' Unpublished report, University of Wollongong, Wollongong.

Voelkl, J.E., Winkelhake, K., Jeffries, J. and Yoshioka, N. (2003) 'Examination of a nursing home environment: are residents engaged in recreation activities?' *Therapeutic Recreation Journal* 37, 4, 300–314.

Warms, C.A., Belza, B.L. and Whitney, J.D. (2007) 'Correlates of physical activity in adults with mobility limitations.' *Family Community Health* 30, 2S, S5–S16.

Weuve, J., Kang, J.H., Manson, J.E., Breteler, M.B., Ware, J.H. and Grodstein, F. (2004) 'Physical activity, including walking and cognitive function in older women.' *Journal of the American Medical Association* 292, 2, 1454–1461.

Williams, S.W., Williams, C.S., Zimmerman, S., Sloane, P.D. *et al.* (2005) 'Characteristics associated with mobility limitation in long-term care residents with dementia.' *The Gerontologist* 45, 1, 62–67.

Woodhead, E.L., Zarit, S.H., Braungart, E.R., Rovine, M.R. and Femia, E.E. (2005) 'Behavioural and psychological symptoms of dementia: the effects of physical activity at adult day care centres.' *Alzheimer's Disorders and Other Dementias* 20, 171–179.

Zeisel, J. (2006) *Inquiry by Design.* New York: W.W. Norton and Co.

Chapter 12

Innovative Dementia Training in the Deep South of the United States

Christopher Jay Johnson and Roxanna H. Johnson

Introduction

In 2002 the Office of Inspector General (OIG) orchestrated a study of training for certified nurse aides (CNAs) working in nursing homes in the United States, and confirmed that in comparison to 15 years previously (i.e. in 1987) current residents were older and sicker; required more assistance with activities of daily living; and took more medications.

It is estimated that roughly 60 to 75 percent of nursing home residents in the US have some type of dementia (Matthews *et al.* 2002). Yet there is a lack of accurate and quality dementia training for CNAs, who provide roughly 90 percent of the hands-on care for residents living in nursing homes (Dodson and Zincavage 2007). The current training for CNAs has not kept pace with the changing care needs of the residents (Jones 2005). Most CNA training is based on the medical model, which places emphasis on physical needs – often ignoring emotional, intellectual, and social needs of the residents (Foner 1994). There is a shortage of practical skills training on the management of dementia and cognitive disorders. The gap in knowledge challenges CNAs to provide quality resident care in working with special resident populations (Lopez 2006).

In response to training needs, we started a consultancy company to provide research-based gerontological and dementia-specific staff training and consultancy for long-term care (LTC) settings. Louisiana is one of the most impoverished and racially divided regions in the US. This results in situations where primarily Caucasians manage and train minority staff in nursing homes. There are key issues of low pay, devalued and stigmatized work, and lack of trust to overcome.

This chapter reports on innovative approaches that were culturally relevant for minority CNAs who cared for and supported people with dementia. We utilized proven learning methods from multiple disciplines in novel ways. This allowed us to incorporate strategies that were applicable to CNAs' lives beyond dementia care. The authors' fundamental principles for training were to have unconditional positive regard for each CNA and encourage them to promote the concept of citizenship for the residents (Rogers 1980). The principles of personhood and its implications for full citizenship were woven into CNA training and then CNAs applied these principles to the care of persons with dementia. In this context, citizenship can be defined as the provision of full rights, liberty, equality, and self-determination free from stigmatization (Boyle 2008). This training team employed Carl Rogers' (1959) methods to establish rapport and develop positive genuine relationships with the care staff. Applying Adlerian concepts in training provided new understandings of behaviors that were transferable knowledge for the care staff to improve dementia care for the residents, and parenting skills.

Our training strategies aimed to empower and reward care workers while offering engaging learning experiences. Spiritually based dementia training provided existential meaning to our lives and the lives of many CNAs as well. Most of the knowledge was purposely transferable for the CNAs' work world and personal family life.

We argue that there were residual benefits as a result of parallel training. Central to cultural differences and dementia care, the trainers' goals were building trust while infusing into the training the idea of the 'oneness of humankind'. There are benefits in using multidimensional strategies to enhance learning and build better communication, trust and relationships with staff and families of people with dementia. Such philosophy and training approaches encouraged better race relations within and outside the nursing home – effectively crossing color lines that often seem immutable in the Deep South.

The South and Black CNAs

In America, racism, patriarchy, and social class serve as interlocking systems of oppression and privilege (Griffin and Hargis 2008; Landry and Platt-Jendrek 1978). Prejudice runs deep among Blacks, Creole, and Whites in the Deep South. As trainers, we understand that many habitual ways in which CNAs perceive the world are shaped by their past experiences. Black women have historically been economically exploited under the repressive systems in the South (Beal 2008; Elkins 1976; Jones 1985). Negative race relations for Black women have been incorporated into their social history and identities (Landry and Platt-Jendrek 1978). Stereotypes, myths, and stigmas concerning race change over time but scars appear to be a well-entrenched feature of America, notably in the South. Black females continue to be disproportionately represented among those on the bottom rung of income and occupational ladders. Living in poverty and raising children without positive participating male family members is a prevalent theme (DeNavas-Walt, Proctor and Smith 2007; Tellis-Nayak and Tellis-Nayak 1989). Most Black CNAs were raised in matriarchies, having little or no relationships with their fathers. As they became adults, most became single parents – a status correlated with poverty in the United States (Glenn, Nock and Waite 2002). In the Deep South, there is a growing low-wage, female, and increasingly non-White workforce composed primarily of Black women. So the long-term care industry in the upcoming decades will see more minority women workers.

Mismatched worlds

In a study of Black nurse aides, Ball *et al.* (2009, p.43) found that in general the workers attributed racism to nursing home residents' historical experience in the South, referring to them as being 'still trapped back in those days'. One CNA that Ball *et al.* (2009, p.41) quote says, 'Race, man, yeah throughout the whole building, it's nothing but Caucasian people that live here. The only people that work here are African Americans. So you know, that ought to tell you something about this facility.' The mismatched world of Black CNAs can be juxtaposed with that of the people they serve. For the most part, the management and nursing home residents and their families are from White middle- to upper-class worlds (Ball *et al.* 2009), while Black CNAs typically live in lower-class families (Beal 2008). Many of these women have children and live in poverty in tumultuous family lives (Beal 2008; Tellis-Nayak and Tellis-Nayak 1989). Most Black births occur out of wedlock (Foster 2008), and these women place greater emphasis on help from extended kinship (e.g. grandparents, mothers, aunts, and children) and less emphasis on marital relationships. In 2008, 40.6 percent of births in the US occurred out of wedlock, with Blacks being America's highest at 72.3 percent. The poverty rate for married couples was dramatically lower than that of single-headed households, even when compared to the rate for single parents with the same education level (Foster 2008). Marriage drops the odds of being poor by 80 percent, with the same effect in terms of reducing one's poverty as adding five to six years of education (Duffy 2005; Foster 2008). According to Lamanna and Reidmann (2008) nearly all life experiences are influenced by economics, and the following factors add stress to poor working women's lives:

1. Most poor working women are more likely to live in government-subsidized housing.

2. They are more likely to have irregular working hours, in minimum or less than minimum wage jobs.

3. Working full-time at minimum wage does not earn enough money to place the family above poverty.

4. Many mothers face problems with job, day care, and transportation availability.

5. Meanwhile children in poverty are more likely to be disabled or chronically ill.

6. These children are more likely to have emotional and behavioral problems than children from families above the poverty line.

7. Due to a lack of education, parenting skills are more likely to be deficient, placing emphasis on corporal punishment.

Work and domestic-related stress

Ejaz *et al.* (2008) isolated three individual-level predictors of job satisfaction for dementia care workers as:

- background characteristics
- personal stressors
- job-related stressors.

With Black CNAs as the lowest-paid workers in the health care labor force, financial and family worries are likely to be personal sources of stress (Stone and Weiner 2001; Tellis-Nayak and Tellis-Nayak 1989). CNA turnover rates are an indication of a degree of unhappiness and are triggered by a variety of factors, among which are job dissatisfaction (Castle, Degenholtz and Rosen 2006; Institute of Medicine 2001; National Commission on Nursing Workforce for Long-Term Care 2005). Typical causes of job stress and workplace dissatisfaction for CNAs relate to:

- low wages and lack of benefits
- poor training
- lack of communication and teamwork
- inadequate supervision

- understaffing

- lack of supplies.

(Parmelee, Laszlo and Taylor 2009)

Intensifying these issues were often race-related interpersonal conflicts among nursing home staff, cliquishness, and incidences of verbal and physical fights (Parmelee *et al.* 2009).

Berdes and Eckert (2007) studied the effects of racial differences between nursing home residents and CNAs, finding that three-quarters of the nurse aides experienced racism on the job. Specifically, one-third of residents exhibited race-related attitudes toward Black CNAs in two ways: racist language (e.g. the 'n' word or 'darkie') and 'malignant racism' where residents hate Blacks and refuse to allow them in their space. Adding to the stigmas of working in LTC, management frequently devalue their work as well. For example, while the authors were conducting training with the manager (part owner) and Black nurse aides, during the feedback session an aide complained about her low pay. The manager replied, 'Well, you can always go work at McDonald's down the street, they're hiring!'. Such comments were common, showing how little some owners or managers valued their Black workers' labor (Berdes and Eckert 2007).

For the CNA, encountering racism is stressful. This is compounded by daily negative encounters with often critical residents and families (Beck *et al.* 1999). Symbolically, the CNA role is to interact with residents like 'family', while avoiding families that are racist or critical, but telling such family members what they want to hear. The Black CNAs must conduct 'face-work' in an attempt not to overstep accepted boundaries, and foster an image or ritual order as it applies to managers and families (Goffman 1963).

Factoring out the top six barriers to job performance, Parmelee *et al.* (2009) identified 'exclusion' as the greatest concern. Exclusion involved CNAs' perceptions of being under-used, under-supervised, and excluded from nursing home communication and decision-making. The strongest independent predictor of job satisfaction was the CNAs' stress-related perception of having no input into care decisions and no feedback about their job performance. This predictor was inconsistent with our observations, which are representative of Black females as having sole responsibility for their families.

Black CNAs' coping mechanisms for stress

Racism and insults directed by White residents toward Black CNAs alters their 'strategies, relationships and outcomes' (Ball *et al.* 2009, p.41). Likewise,

Ball *et al.* (2009, p.43) quote a Black CNA who says, 'At times, when they [the residents] throw out the n-word. I have been in this field so long I don't get upset and irate like some staff have.' Black CNAs used dementia as the determining factor of whether they accepted or rejected prejudiced residents. If residents had dementia they had an excuse, but if not, they were responsible for their bigotry and the aides tended to avoid them (Ball *et al.* 2009).

Historically, poor women have been called upon to reveal personal information about themselves and their families in order to receive means-tested government support. Dodson and Schmalzbauer (2005, p.949) argue that poor mothers tended to conceal their personal lives in response to punitive authorities and stigmatization. In line with this, Braithwaite, Taylor and Treadwell (2009) point out that Black women under-utilize mental health services, believing in the stereotype of Black women as being strong enough to overcome anything. Yet, self-reported racism is correlated with mental ill health such as negative moods and depression (Brondolo *et al.* 2008).

Dodson and Zincavage's (2007) research of CNAs found that when nursing homes drew on family ideology at work it promoted good care of residents. While their study found that carers valued fictitious kinship with residents, they also suspected that the 'family model' was used to exploit these low-income CNAs. Reflecting a subordinate and racial version of being 'part of the family', Dodson and Zincavage call for change: first, through an ethic of reciprocity, and second, they call for concrete changes towards placing equal value on the humanity of both those who need care and of those who give care!

Nursing home studies indicate that satisfaction gained from affective ties with residents serves to counterbalance the more negative aspects of care work and increase retention (Ball *et al.* 2009). Berdes and Eckert (2007) discuss the idea of 'fictive kinship' where CNAs use family metaphors to describe the care of residents, using their own family experiences of care. Yet the CNAs frequently fail to get the same genuine regard from the owners and/or families. Therefore one of our training strategies was to emphasize the rewarding aspects of their work. Coping with stigma and low status is attached to the job. Black CNAs try to trade their experiences of objective (economic, legal, political) oppression for subjective (moral, ethical, philosophical) superiority as part of their lifetime experience (Ball *et al.* 2009, p.46).

In order to manage stress, Black women are more likely to use the most detrimental forms of passive coping, such as avoidance and denial (Noh and Kaspar 2003), which are linked to high blood pressure while talking about problems improves blood pressure (Smyth and Yarandi 1996). The approaches to coping with stress vary according to people's beliefs and resources. Yet Noh and Kaspar (2003) indicate that Black CNAs opt for emotion-focused strategies of removing themselves from stressors, rather than choosing problem-focused approaches. Emotion-focused coping is a type of avoidance, while problem-focused coping is analogous to dealing with problems directly and coping well (Scott and House 2005; Utsey, Adams and Bolden 2000). Research indicates a relationship between avoidance coping, denial, and greater distress. While avoidance is an emotion-focused reaction to situations, it ultimately fails to alleviate problems (Scott and House 2005). In light of this, it became clear that another key training strategy was to introduce better methods of coping with stress and provide Black CNAs with a place and permission to vent their emotions.

Obstacles and barriers between the Black CNA and Caucasian trainers

There are multifaceted barriers that often operate simultaneously between the Black CNAs and White trainers. These features can serve as obstacles both to their receptivity to the trainers as persons and to internalization of their educational approaches to person-centered dementia care. The following are some salient differences in the social worlds of Black CNAs and White trainers which must be acknowledged in order to achieve the goal of person-centered training.

Cultural differences

There are usually cultural differences between trainers and CNAs beyond the obvious. Attitudes in the consulting business have been shaped by our inter-racial family, multicultural religion (Baha'i Faith), and inter-racial friendships. Yet we still do not totally understand the social world of Black CNAs. Although CNAs were reluctant to share their world, when we shared prejudices that were aimed toward us it helped to promote understandings and built a bridge between us, since they had experienced similar challenges.

Economic differences

The daily economic woes of Black CNAs are ubiquitous. Add to this the fact that many managers we have encountered rarely offer the nurse aides a free meal or meals at a reduced rate, while working for minimum wage. This alone is hard to fathom. Providing meals at a reduced rate with appropriate scheduled break times would seem to be a necessity, but was frequently overlooked in nursing homes.

Educational barriers

To break down the barriers in educational differences we asked the CNAs to call us by our first names, to do away with elitism. We also instilled the idea that knowledge is power and something that no one can ever take away from them. In this case, we aspired to provide CNAs with knowledge of techniques which would make their work world and home life more manageable.

Parenting barriers

Black CNAs' parenting skills tend to place much higher emphasis on corporal punishment. These methods are entrenched in the culture of the Black working poor. As part of the training, we use Alfred Adler's (1931) approach to understanding the causes for behaviors. The Adlerian model identifies and highlights the 'goal' of behaviors that challenge carers and/or parents. These new insights are extremely effective for modifying behaviors of all people. This style of cross-training was very much appreciated and offered new coping strategies for Black CNAs.

Lack of encouragement

We distinguish democratic versus autocratic methods of communicating. Emphasizing person-centered care for people with dementia, we point out encouragement as a primary form of reinforcement, placing the residents as active agents essential to citizenship. Specific strategies are used to focus on people's unique assets and strengths to build self-confidence and self-worth. Such tactics focus on seeing positive characteristics in the residents. In addition, the CNAs learn to value the individuality of the person with dementia; not to make acceptance dependent on the person's cooperative behaviors; and to have faith in the person with dementia, so that they will come to believe in themselves. Such attitude changes can reduce feelings of powerlessness and inadequacy (Berdes and Eckert 2007). Encouragement is given for effort or improvement, to shape targeted behaviors.

The shifts in discourses positioning people with dementia as active agents are paramount. The most powerful forces in human relationships are expectations. The CNAs quickly learn that they can influence a person's behavior by changing their own expectations. This requires the belief that it can happen, the faith that it will, and reasonable (not unreasonable) standards of expectations. Some CNAs give up on people with dementia, feeling hopeless, and then instill hopelessness further by doing everything for them. We teach Black CNAs to avoid using discouraging words and actions, and instead to tell the person what they *can do* rather than what they cannot do.

When there is low pay, find meaningful rewards

How do you motivate someone to learn when they are being paid minimum wage? The obvious disincentives of low pay can create lethargy. Training can be likened to another disruption in daily routines, being short-handed, and trying to accomplish insurmountable work. Additionally, you have a Caucasian couple coming in to pontificate dementia facts. Initially some Black CNAs were friendly and some were indifferent. The low pay, stigmatization of their role and work, and the lack of appreciation that many feel from the management were disincentives to learn something in mandatory in-service training. To counter cynical attitudes with positive ones we brought the CNAs gifts that were raffled off at the end of training as a reward for participation. We also brought seasonal fresh fruit and talked about healthy lifestyles, because CNAs rarely get anything free, depending upon the facility. They were very grateful for the positive reinforcement, and these strategies help to establish relationships.

Bridging gaps between black and white

Some aides view the trainers as either irrelevant to understanding their work world, or as a threat to them. In order to deal with such thoughts or emotions, a few CNAs present the persona of the proverbial 'know-it-all' where everything the trainers say is obvious to them. Others might feel threatened by persons trained in gerontology, or by their race, and consequently become adversarial. Some feel they might be exposed for doing things incorrectly and be looked down upon. CNAs experiencing such threats used avoidance by not being present either bodily or in mind (e.g. strategies that include 'talking while he is talking', sleeping, not paying attention, showing up late or just not showing up). Many Black CNAs have little social interaction with White trainers and/or display a general lack of trust based on a lifetime of negative experiences with White authority figures. Our consulting company utilized a series of pedagogical strategies to address the issues discussed thus far. These are set out below.

1. PERSON-CENTERED TRAINING

Reflective listening and having unconditional positive regard for CNAs as an approach to training was critical. Making an effort to learn names, asking for feedback, and listening to complaints about life are part of being person-centered. Carl Rogers (1980), the author of person-centered therapy, influences us to want Black CNAs to self-actualize. We show genuine caring, interest, and compassion for all CNAs as persons free of stigmas. Our view emphasizes that we are all one race, the human race. Many Black CNAs are often marginal to the mainline public, families of residents, residents, or owners of facilities in the Deep South (Foner 1994). Most have unique names or other presentations of self, and receiving 'unconditional positive regard' (Rogers 1980) from the trainers was necessary. Rogers believed that 'conditional positive regard' leads to 'conditions of worth', which, in turn, can lead to alienation from true feelings and so to anxiety and threat, which blocks self-actualization. We indicated our appreciation of the CNAs as carers and persons, when few in their world take time to do this. We always saw the CNAs as persons, and this was at the core of our approach to establishing meaningful relationships.

2. WORK AS WORSHIP

We frequently told the CNAs, as a fundamental principle of training, that their work was special, spiritually based, and would earn them a 'high place in Heaven' for the services they rendered. Most CNAs liked this and openly displayed appreciation by nodding their heads when this was said. The managers we have worked with, with few exceptions, rarely acknowledge their work in that way.

3. MUTUAL SHARING

We shared some information about our own lives and families from time to time; this made us human. When opportunity knocked, we showed interest in whatever each Black CNA might have wanted to share about her personal life. Although Black CNAs often tightly managed such sharing until trust was there, our approach was to listen, being non-judgmental. The possibility for developing relationships was also open during informal chats on breaks when CNAs would share information about their personal lives. As White trainers from different cultures and backgrounds we had to find creative ways to connect and develop trust. One such strategy was to share our personal frailties, illnesses, maladies, and life challenges with them.

4. ACKNOWLEDGING UNITY THROUGH DIVERSITY

There are pressures of idealized conduct with marginalized people in special workplaces. The lower class in America regularly deviate (in appearance, language, and behavior) from middle- and upper middle-class norms, which can lead to stigmatization (Gilbert 2002). For example, some of these women wore dreadlocks, long fake nails, extravagant wigs and hair extensions, and tattoos. From our experiences living in the South, such presentations of self are often viewed as discreditable by dominant White management and families. While the management attempted to teach CNAs the importance of 'impression management', there was often resistance because of the lack of relationships (Goffman 1963, p.42). With White families and residents, Black CNAs often attempt to learn to talk and act White while following the prescribed norms. We would periodically discuss some CNAs' subsequent feelings of ambivalence and alienation that could emerge from such normative expectations.

Earning minimum wage with no health insurance and receiving very small raises when they were loyal employees was not reassuring. Many of the CNAs we worked with were frustrated about their pay, working without sufficient staff, and the little time they had to spend with the residents. The training sessions were a vehicle for some venting, but it is important to conduct this prudently and avoid 'gripe' sessions.

We often discussed racist remarks that residents made and outlined strategies on how to deal with them. Having lived a life of racism within a racist Southern Culture, the residents with dementia often make little attempt to modify their behavior; so the approach to learn was how to cope by changing the subject or sometimes just ignoring it. Hurtful remarks were meant to hurt the Black CNAs, so the strategy we proposed from the Adlerian approach was to not act hurt (allowing the prejudiced person to achieve their goal). This by no means excluded the strategy of asking the residents to please stop using the 'n' word!

5. Cousinhood of humankind

In our approach to relationships, we quickly established the fact that we (the entire human race) are all at least fifty-second cousins, a fact that was brought out by anthropological researcher Murchie (1978) in his book *The Seven Mysteries of Life*. Dodson and Zincavage cite one CNA's thoughts about her connection to her residents:

> The same way I think about my mother, this is the same way I'm thinking about these residents. I consider them like they are my own. But it's a very hard job, we don't get paid enough for the job, and sometimes you feel like every day you do more and more and more, and the money is less. (Dodson and Zincavage 2007, p.1)

6. Humility and simplicity

Since most Black CNAs are not highly educated, it is not a good idea for trainers to use phrases such as 'catastrophic behavior', referring to angry outbursts as is common in many training manuals. It was important to be humble and not think that because we had more education we were superior. Instead, our thoughts were that CNAs had numerous experiences and learning was mutual. During training it was not unusual for us to ask them what strategies they used that worked best.

7. COLLABORATIVE PROJECTS BETWEEN STAFF AND TRAINERS

Based upon an idea from a Canadian nursing home, we had the CNAs work to assist in the construction of a large 'activity calendar' that used pictures of the CNAs' children and grandchildren to connect their families to the workplace. We also had the CNAs lead us in designing a picture logo for their nursing home's philosophy of care. The logo was then developed into posters that were hung throughout the facility. Then the logo was developed further into badges used to hold their name tags. This process encouraged the CNAs to have input and ownership. A voice and a choice are invaluable when used appropriately.

In one nursing home, we worked with Black CNAs to give the shower and bathing room a home-like makeover. The CNAs who worked daily on the dementia neighborhood and were responsible for residents' bathing were asked to participate. They were very eager to get involved and given a budget, guidelines, and the time to purchase make-over items. This was empowering and encouraged the CNAs to be a part of the process and change. The physical changes were significant, but more important were the positive changes in the CNAs' attitudes. For example, after this project was over, in our view they were twice as receptive to our training. Also, they would offer suggestions for further improvements to the dementia neighborhood.

8. INCORPORATING MULTIPLE LEARNING
TECHNIQUES TO CAPTIVATE CNAs

Yamada (2002) points out that the typical CNA in America is female and between the ages of 18 and 44 (over 90 percent). Most have finished high school but few have formal education beyond that or are able to further their current education. These demographics and work conditions for nursing home CNAs highlight little change over the intervening years.

In designing training we address the following:

- who we are training

- their age

- gender

- culture

- level of education

- dementia knowledge.

As well as this, we recognize and appreciate that people have different learning styles. The three basic types of learning styles (Vincent and Ross 2001) are:

- *Visual learners* learn by watching. Their brain recalls images from the past when trying to remember and can picture the way things look in their mind.

- *Auditory learners* learn by listening and remember facts when presented in the form of a reading or discussion, a poem, song, or melody. Sometimes auditory learners have trouble reading because they do not visualize well.

- *Kinesthetic learners* learn best by hands-on learning and role playing. They learn by doing and are interested in exploring how things work and are often successful in jobs that provide creative outlets.

In addition to the above, part of the multilearning strategies we incorporated into CNA training were:

- *role playing*, where carers were asked to play the role of the person with dementia in order to comprehend certain realities of care

- *case studies* used to reinforce points that had been made, sometimes with pictures or stories

- *discussion groups* among the CNAs, where they discussed intervention strategies

- *problem-solving sessions*, where they were given a problem to solve through group or individual participation

- *sensory deprivation exercises*, where the CNAs were given supplies to mimic age-related sensory deprivations in order to foster better empathy and understanding of the residents

- *Adlerian training techniques* that provided new methods of identifying the goals of behaviors as a part of the dementia training.

These applications parallel procedures for parenting.

9. Linking commonalities

In training we emphasized the personhood of both the residents and staff, evaluating what they have in common. It was important to have short biographies of each resident to describe their distinctive lives, special interests, and qualities. Such information allowed the CNAs to discover each resident's life history and encouraged bonding based on commonalities. While problem-solving, we used the biographical information to explore:

- past occupations
- hobbies
- family members such as parents and siblings
- memorable experiences
- recognition of special accomplishments.

This information was used to unpick what the CNAs might have perceived as a problem behavior that ultimately was a life-long habit that needed a fresh perspective. The nurse aides learned to embrace residents' unique behaviors rather than resist.

Management and empowering Black CNAs

Many economic and psychological theories depict management and owners of nursing homes as slaves to self-interest (Gass 2005). The for-profit market dominates the nursing home industry and has been lucratively profitable (Polivka-West and Okano 2008). More fair, just, and sustainable schemes will need to be explored to offer better pay and respect for CNAs. These ideals have too often been dismissed as naive. The transition to fair pay, and elevation of the CNAs' value and status of the work they do, will present great challenges for nursing home owners. Achieving this will require a transformation in thought and action for the leaders of the nursing home industry. The cultural forces at play are powerful and demand re-examination if we are to move forward. Black CNAs clearly differentiate various barriers, but the consensus is that low pay, status, devalued work, heavy workload, and lack of teamwork are the most problematic.

Conclusions

We have delineated the need for unique approaches to training minority Black CNAs in the Deep South of the US. Special issues that warrant attention for this group included racism, mismatched work worlds, domestic stressors, and lack of positive coping mechanisms. Key strategies for changing the predicament of Black CNAs focused on emphasizing the rewarding aspects of their jobs and introducing new coping strategies.

The blending of better interpersonal communication skills and conflict management was well received by Black CNAs. Adlerian concepts were employed to increase intrinsic job satisfaction coupled with feelings of empowerment. The dual training approaches advocated in this chapter offered new knowledge for understanding the goals of behavior for all people. The person-centered training techniques were central to care and also fostered citizenship of the people with dementia. Our methods of training helped staff create beneficence both for the people with dementia and for the CNAs' own family members. There is a need for wider applications of some of these ideas to influence current theories and promote better race relations in the nursing home, especially in the Deep South in America. Moreover, we hope this chapter will be a springboard for more extensive research into bridging racial barriers both in training and staff management in long-term care, to promote better dementia care.

References

Adler, A. (1931) *What Life Could Mean to You*. Center City, MN: Hazelden.

Ball, M., Lepore, M., Perkins, M., Hollingsworth, C. and Sweatman, M. (2009) '"They are the reason I come to work": the meaning of resident–staff relationships in assisted living.' *Journal of Aging Studies* 23, 37–47.

Barlett, R. and O'Connor, D. (2011) 'Broadening the Dementia Debate: Towards Social Citizenship.' *British Journal of Social Work 41*, 1: 192–193.

Beal, F.M. (2008) 'Double Jeopardy: To Be Black and Female.' In G.S. Wilmore and J.H. Cone (eds) *Black Theology: A Documentary History, 1966–1979*. Maryknoll: Orbis Books.

Beck, C., Ortigara, A., Mercer, S. and Shue, V. (1999) 'Enabling and empowering certified nursing assistants for quality dementia care.' *International Journal of Geriatric Psychiatry 14*, 197–212.

Berdes, C. and Eckert, J. (2007) 'The language of caring: nurse aides' use of family metaphors conveys affective care.' *The Gerontologist 47*, 3, 340–349.

Boyle, G. (2008) 'The Mental Capacity Act 2005: promoting the citizenship of people with dementia?' *Health and Social Care in the Community 16*, 5, 529–537.

Brondolo, E., Libby, D., Denton, E., Thompson, S. *et al.* (2008) 'Racism and ambulatory blood pressure in a community sample.' *Psychosomatic Medicine 70*, 49–56.

Braithwaite, R., Taylor, S. and Treadwell, H. (2009) *Health Issues in the Black Community*. New York: Jossey-Bass.

Castle, N., Degenholtz, H. and Rosen, J. (2006) 'Determinants of staff job satisfaction of caregivers in two nursing homes in Pennsylvania.' *BMC Health Services Research*. Available at www.biomedcentral.com/1472-6963/6/60, accessed on 20 July 2009.

DeNavas-Walt, C., Proctor, B.D. and Smith, J. (2007) *Current Population Reports, Series P60–233. Income, Poverty and Health Insurance Coverage in the United States: 2006*. Washington, DC: US Census Bureau.

Dodson, L. and Schmalzbauer, L. (2005) 'Poor women and habits of hiding: participatory methods in poverty research.' *Journal of Marriage and Family 67*, 4, 949–959.

Dodson, L. and Zincavage, R. (2007) '"It's like a family": caring labor, exploitation, and race in nursing homes.' *Gender and Society 21*, 905–928.

Duffy, M. (2005) 'Reproducing labour inequalities: challenges for feminists conceptualizing care at the intersections of gender, race, and class.' *Gender and Society 19*, 1, 66–82.

Ejaz, F., Noelker, L., Menne, H. and Bagaka, J. (2008) 'The impact of stress and support on direct care workers' job satisfaction.' *The Gerontologist 48*, 1, 60–70.

Elkins, S. (1976) *Slavery: A Problem in American Institutional and Intellectual Life*, 3rd edition. Chicago, IL: University of Chicago Press.

Foner, N. (1994) *The Caregiving Dilemma: Work in an American Nursing Home*. Berkeley, CA: University of California Press.

Foster, F. (2008) *Love and Marriage in Early African America*. Boston, MA: Northeastern University Press.

Gass, T. (2005) *Nobody's Home: Candid Reflections of a Nursing Home Aide*. New York: Cornell University Press.

Gilbert, D. (2002) *The American Class Structure*. New York: Wadsworth.

Glenn, N.D., Nock, S.L. and Waite, L.J. (2002) *Why Marriage Matters: Twenty-One Conclusions from the Social Sciences*. New York: Institute for American Values.

Goffman, E. (1963) *Stigma: Notes on the Management of Spoiled Identity*. New York: Prentice-Hall.

Griffin, L. and Hargis, P. (2008) 'Still distinctive after all these years: trends in racial attitudes in and out of the South.' *Southern Culture 14*, 3, 117–141.

Institute of Medicine (2001) *Improving the Quality of Long-Term Care.* Washington, DC: National Academy Press.

Jones, J. (1985) *Labor of Love, Labor of Sorrow.* New York: Basic Books.

Jones, J. (2005) 'Writing Women's History: What's Feminism Got to Do With It?' In C. Berkin, J.L. Pinch and C.S. Appel (eds) *Exploring Women's Studies: Looking Forward, Looking Back.* New York: Prentice-Hall.

Lamanna, M. and Reidmann, A. (2008) *Marriages and Families: Making Choices in a Diverse Society.* New York: Wadsworth Publishing.

Landry, B. and Platt-Jendrek, M. (1978) 'The empowerment of wives in middle-class black families.' *Journal of Marriage and Family 40*, 4, 787–797.

Lopez, S. (2006) 'Culture change management in long-term care: a shop-floor view.' *Politics and Society 43*, 1, 55–79.

Matthews, F., Dening, T. and the UK Medical Research Council Cognitive Function and Ageing Study (2002) 'The prevalence of dementia in institutional care.' *The Lancet 360*, 9328, 225–226.

Murchie, G. (1978) *The Seven Mysteries of Life.* New York: Houghton Mifflin.

National Commission on Nursing Workforce for Long-Term Care (2005) *Act Now: For Your Tomorrow.* Available at www.ahcancal.org/research_data/staffing/Documents/Nursing_Workforce_Report. pdf, accessed on 10 November 2011.

Noh, S. and Kaspar, V. (2003) 'Perceived discrimination and depression: moderating the effects of coping, acculturation and ethnic support.' *American Journal of Public Health 93*, 2, 232–238.

Office of Inspector General (2002) *Nurse Aide Training.* Washington, DC: US Department of Health and Human Services.

Parmelee, P.A., Laszlo, M.C. and Taylor, J.A. (2009) 'Perceived barriers to effective job performance among nursing assistants in long-term care.' *Journal of the American Medical Directors Association 10*, 8, 559–567.

Polivka-West, L. and Okano, K. (2008) 'Nursing home regulation and quality assurance in the States: seeking greater effectiveness for better care.' *Generations 32*, 3, 62–66.

Rogers, C. (1959) 'A Theory of Therapy, Personality and Interpersonal Relationships as Developed in the Client-Centered Framework.' In S. Koch (ed.) *Psychology: A Study of a Science. Vol. 3: Formulations of the Person and the Social Context.* New York: McGraw.

Rogers, C. (1980) *A Way of Being.* Boston: Houghton Mifflin.

Scott, L.D. Jr. and House, L.E. (2005) 'Relationship of distress and perceived control to coping with perceived racial discrimination among black youth.' *The Journal of Black Psychology 31*, 3, 254–272.

Smyth, K. and Yarandi, H.N. (1996) 'Factor analysis of the ways of coping questionnaire for African-American women.' *Nursing Research 45*, 1, 25–29.

Stone, R.I. and Weiner, J.M. (2001) *Who Will Care for Us?* Washington, DC: Urban Institute and the American Association of Homes and Services for the Aging.

Tellis-Nayak, V. and Tellis-Nayak, M. (1989) 'Quality of care and the burden of two cultures: when the world of the nurse's aide enters the world of the nursing home.' *The Gerontologist 29*, 3, 307–313.

Utsey, S.O., Adams, E.P. and Bolden, M. (2000) 'Development and initial validation of the Africultural coping systems inventory.' *The Journal of Black Psychology 26*, 2, 194–215.

Vincent, A. and Ross, D. (2001) 'Personalize training: determine learning styles, personality types and multiple intelligences online.' *The Learning Organization 8*, 1, 36–43.

Yamada, Y. (2002) 'Profile of home care aides, nursing home aides, and hospital aides: historical changes and data recommendations.' *The Gerontologist 42*, 2, 199–206.

Conclusion

Anthea Innes, Fiona Kelly and Louise McCabe

This collection has brought together policy, practice and theorising, and as such reflects key issues in the current context where dementia care is constantly evolving. The collection presents a selection of international theory-based policy and practice contributions and therefore brings together three main strands of work in the dementia studies arena: theory, policy and practice.

Dementia is of interest to national governments mainly due to the financial pressures dementia creates for society. Practitioners are interested in dementia because it poses significant challenges to achieving high-quality care outcomes for their clients. (Even those who have not chosen to specialise in this area are likely to encounter dementia in other areas of practice delivery.) Academics from diverse disciplines have been attracted to dementia as a subject of empirical inquiry reflecting the intellectual appeal of investigating a topic/condition/disease that poses many challenges in terms of conceptualisation, ethical conduct (of both practice and research), structure of targets and measurement of outcomes.

The importance of conceptualising dementia was illustrated in Part I of this book. Innes (Chapter 1) provides an overview of different approaches to understanding and conceptualising dementia that stem from different disciplinary starting points. Innes herself starts from a social science perspective of knowledge to challenge thinking about what particular understandings of dementia could mean for policy, research and practice. Different ways of understanding dementia were then exemplified by Dudgeon (Chapter 2), who uses conceptualisations of dementia that will attract policy makers' attention in a drive for more effective resource allocation and status to be awarded to dementia at a national level. In contrast, Telford, Gallagher and Reynish (Chapter 4) demonstrate the need to ground understandings of dementia in a practice-oriented context to improve the day-to-day care received by those with dementia, using a multitude of components. Coley, Berr and Andrieu (Chapter 3) remind us of the limits of research used to influence medical practices, and of the need for larger-scale research studies that can shape and inform medical decisions and lifestyle choices. Collectively the chapters in Part I of this book illustrate the importance of using models, concepts and ideas about dementia to shape dementia care research, policy and practice. This means that theory is used as a way to influence policy and practice developments, as well as to challenge existing knowledge and generate new ideas that will lead to positive and informed outcomes, both for those who live with dementia and for those who support them.

Future theoretical work in the dementia field needs to build on what is already known about dementia while challenging practices that are based on implicit or partial knowledge that is often presented and used as 'facts'. In this way the study, practice and structures of dementia care can evolve and improve over time.

The case studies in Part II, the policy section of the book, demonstrate how and why dementia-specific policy develops, and provide detail on the specific processes undertaken in each particular place. The policy chapters demonstrate the need for a compelling case to motivate governments to act, but even then, implementation can be challenging. There is a shared aim among the different countries to reduce stigma and improve knowledge and awareness of dementia among the general public. Early and accurate diagnosis with good information and support following diagnosis are also identified as priorities across the chapters in this section of the book. In addition, the provision of good quality care was, unsurprisingly, highlighted. The differences between the case studies relate to the broader political, cultural and social context in each country. England and France have complex and quite different health and social care systems that have been built over many years, which relate to the political, economic and social history in each country. Therefore, Banerjee (Chapter 5) and Guisset-Martinez (Chapter 6) report different specific approaches to improve dementia care and the experiences of people with dementia and their carers. There were clear challenges to implementing the dementia strategies due to financial constraints and also existing, complex and often changing health and social care systems. All chapters demonstrate the commitment and in-depth work of those involved in developing the plans and strategies.

Dementia strategies, as evidenced here, can have a strong impact in the way that they influence thinking among professionals and practitioners and lead to change in practice, as well as providing important support for the further development or expansion of existing services. For the future it seems likely that dementia-specific policy will be supported by increasingly dramatic statistics showing a continued rise in the number of people with dementia, and rising care and treatment costs. However, the future aim for policy should not be about creating new policy, but instead about finding innovative ways to achieve the key aims of existing national strategies within increasingly constrained budgets. It will be interesting to compare how dementia care develops in response to the strategies in different countries; perhaps a small country like Malta will benefit from having a compact system that can be more responsive and quicker to change.

While the chapters in Part III, the practice section, discuss diverse issues (education and training, post-diagnostic support, environmental design) from a range of countries and cultures (America, Australia, India and the United Kingdom), there are several themes which cut across both cultures and practice issues. These are: the ever-present, and increasing, need for a knowledgeable workforce who can in turn teach and support families; the importance of using existing resources, whether it be community networks, volunteers, community buildings or expertise from another discipline to deliver services; the importance of environmental design for promoting good practice and in supporting the person with dementia and caregivers; and the trend towards providing care that suits individual need, whether it be the family carer's needs or the needs of the person with dementia.

It is clear from these chapters that the future of services for people with dementia and their families lies in finding innovative, cost-efficient responses to policy. One way of achieving this, as this collection demonstrates, is the use of local resources – local people with local knowledge, established social networks or existing community buildings (preferably built or adapted using dementia-friendly principles) – to deliver appropriate services as required. Another way is to use the skills of multidisciplinary teams, thus ensuring that expertise is shared and tasks are not duplicated. Another way of ensuring efficient and effective delivery of services is a well-educated workforce, educated in a multidimensional understanding of dementia that recognises the complex (social, psychological, spiritual, physical, institutional and structural) facets of living with dementia and of working to support those affected by dementia. The challenge now is to integrate these pieces of the jigsaw into a coherent, efficient and cost-effective whole in a way that truly meets the needs and wishes of all concerned.

There are five key interrelating themes that appear throughout this collection. They are as follows.

1. Dementia-specific policy

Policy is important, not just to those who develop policy or to those who study and report on the development of policy initiatives, but also to those delivering and receiving care and support. Dudgeon (Chapter 2), Banerjee (Chapter 5) and Scerri (Chapter 8) demonstrate the importance of influencing policy in direct ways, whether this is to lobby national policy makers, or (as in McCabe's example in Chapter 7) to develop local-level policy to support innovation at a regional level. In many countries, policy drivers shape the action taken to develop care practices. Kelly and Szymczynska (Chapter 9) provide an example of how practice is directly shaped and developed by policy drivers and targets in the UK. Policy plays a key role in how care, treatment and support are delivered to people with dementia and their carers. However, in middle- and low-income countries, as illustrated in Chapter 10 by Dias, policy may be less influential, with the development of care and support for people with dementia driven from the local level by committed professionals, practitioners and family carers. As services develop, however, this can lead to a drive to develop policy to raise awareness of key issues about dementia care and provide a more strategic approach to providing care and support. Innes (Chapter 1) argues that holistic models for dementia care require an approach that integrates theory, policy and practice. Developing policy with a clear understanding of the approach being advocated is likely to have a greater positive impact for practice, and consequently the care that people with dementia receive.

2. Early detection and diagnosis

Early detection and diagnosis of dementia is raised within theoretical discussions about dementia and the future of dementia care. The complexities of identifying and moderating risk factors associated with dementia was outlined by Coley, Berr and Andrieu (Chapter 3), while the national dementia strategies discussed by Banerjee (Chapter 5), Guisset-Martinez (Chapter 6) and Scerri (Chapter 8) all drew attention to early identification and diagnosis of dementia. This issue is also discussed by Kelly and Szymczynska (Chapter 9) in relation to the development of practices in two regions of Scotland to bring about early diagnosis and provide high-quality post-diagnostic support. Early diagnosis is a key issue for the future of dementia care, as this provides the opportunity to promote support at an early point in the journey through dementia for people with dementia and their families, which may prevent the need for costly crisis intervention further down the line. Providing psychosocial interventions to promote the abilities of the person with dementia and to provide support for carers may also enable those with dementia to retain abilities for longer and allow for forward planning, should their condition deteriorate.

3. Conceptualising dementia

Conceptualising dementia is a recurrent theme; from Part I, which discusses how different ways of understanding dementia shape theory, policy and practice, to Part II, which discusses the concern of dementia strategies to raise public awareness and reduce the stigma associated with dementia, and Part III, where the authors discuss different approaches to the teaching and training of professionals and care workers to better support people with dementia and their families. In all of these accounts, the key goal is to improve understanding of dementia by all those affected by it, be they people with dementia themselves, their families, those working to support and care for people with dementia and their families, educators and trainers, the general population, and policy and decision makers (see particularly Dias (Chapter 10); deVries and Traynor (Chapter 11); Johnson and Johnson (Chapter 12)). Understanding the progress and prognosis of dementia and the various challenges experienced by people with dementia and those who support and care for them is crucial for the development and delivery of services that are appropriate, meaningful and valued by those in receipt of them (see Kelly and Szymczynska (Chapter 9) and Dias (Chapter 10)). This collection has identified examples of innovative ways of achieving this, and it is hoped that these approaches can be replicated in a range of countries and care settings.

4. The views of people with dementia

This collection of chapters focuses on the experience of caring from professionals' viewpoints (McCabe (Chapter 7); Kelly and Szymczynska (Chapter 9); Johnson and Johnson (Chapter 12)) and the experience of living with dementia from the perspectives of people with dementia themselves and their family carers (Banerjee (Chapter 5); McCabe (Chapter 7); Kelly and Szymczynska (Chapter 9)). The importance of different viewpoints is discussed for the evaluation of services and the development of policy, including national dementia strategies. Consulting with people with dementia is now widely practised in high-quality research into their experiences and is replacing proxy accounts previously considered sufficient to establish an evidence base. People with dementia and their family members should be consulted on such important issues as the direction and focus of policy and the type of services to be provided, and there are ever-increasing moves to include stakeholder views. However, as this collection illustrates, accounts of service provision and aspirations for policy indicate the gulf that sometimes exists between policy and practice and between practice and people's everyday experiences. For example, Kelly and Szymczynska (Chapter 9) identify family carers' recognition that if their family member has been diagnosed with a dementia other than Alzheimer's disease (i.e. vascular dementia) they received little or no follow-up from professionals following their diagnosis. This suggests a practice bias in favour of Alzheimer's disease, to the detriment and potential isolation of people with a different type of dementia, and their families. Using another lens to view an issue can therefore be a fruitful way to interrogate it; learning from such viewpoints to develop equitable services is the next challenge.

5. Innovation and change

Throughout the book authors highlight the need for change and innovation within dementia care. It is clear that current provision of treatment, care and support for people with dementia and their carers is not always adequate, and this is a view common in all the different countries discussed in the book. Innes (Chapter 1), Dudgeon (Chapter 2) and Telford, Gallagher and Reynish (Chapter 4) explore different ways of understanding dementia and call for new thinking about dementia as a mechanism to promote change and improvement in the way care is provided for people with dementia.

All the dementia strategies described call for significant change in the way dementia care is delivered and promote innovation as the way forward. Coley, Berr and Andrieu (Chapter 3) highlight potential avenues for innovation within biomedical approaches to care and treatment for dementia and approaches to prevention and treatment. Similarly, Kelly and Szymczynska (Chapter 9), Dias (Chapter 10), deVries and Traynor (Chapter 11) and Johnson and Johnson (Chapter 12) all highlight innovative approaches and interventions aimed at supporting people with dementia and their carers and report the successes of these. Dias's work is particularly innovative. Here, local care workers work closely with family members to identify strategies unique to each family to support them to care for the person with dementia at home. While this might seem labour-intensive to implement on a large scale, and recruitment and retention of care workers might be challenging, it is an intuitively appealing approach that might help resolve some of the difficulties currently experienced by people with dementia and their family members (inconsistent home care services, isolation or burden) and by those providing care (burnout or stress). This work also has several other functions: it raises awareness within the community about dementia through teaching and mentoring local care workers (and by doing so, we may hope, reduces some of the stigma and fear attached to dementia); it uses local knowledge and local people to offer support to family members who are struggling to cope with a relative with dementia at home; and it ensures cascading of knowledge to immediate and extended family members. In this way, with minimal financial outlay, it capitalises on the availability of local resources (local people) to fill an identified gap in service provision for people with dementia and their family members. In times of cutbacks and increasingly limited resources, this is an approach which could be transferred to communities beyond India (Chapter 10) and could also be a way to address some of the goals of national dementia strategies.

In another example of the use of existing resources in innovative ways, Kelly and Szymczynska (Chapter 9) identify how working across disciplines can result in more cohesive delivery of services. This is particularly useful in memory services, where diagnosis requires input from fields such as psychology, psychiatry, social work and occupational therapy. Here the resource being used is the skill and expertise of other professionals, and this also, in straitened economic times, would seem to be a logical approach to ensure delivery of consistent and timely support to people with dementia and their families.

An area receiving increasing global attention is the importance of environmental design in either supporting or undermining independence or well-being of the people with dementia, whether in the home or in care. This is discussed by Dias (Chapter 10) and deVries and Traynor (Chapter 11). deVries and Traynor focus on the ways design can support or diminish mobility and activity levels of people with dementia in a care home, while Dias reports that one of the areas in which the care workers support family members caring for a person with dementia at home is through advising on modifying, in simple ways, the design of the house to make it less confusing and safer for the person with dementia, thereby aiming to reduce the stress of the family carer. In these two chapters, environmental design and practice intersect; each influences the other in either promoting or inhibiting innovation and good practice and in promoting or undermining the well-being of people with dementia and those who support and care for them. This is an area that is attracting increasing attention in practice, policy, building design and architecture; the challenge now is to integrate innovations and ideas across multidisciplinary fields and ensure that each field's expertise informs the others. While the current focus is on maintaining independence and maximising abilities, future work should also focus on ensuring that environmental design meets the needs of people with dementia who are nearing the end of their lives; this is a neglected area in practice and research.

The future of theoretically informed policy and practice?

As this edited collection demonstrates, there are many ways to support people with dementia and their families, namely through a theoretically informed understanding of what dementia is and what the experience of this might be, policy directives to support practice and care experiences, and innovations across the globe to promote high-quality care in practice. This collection demonstrates that contemporary innovations are centring on available resources rather than developing new initiatives requiring new funding; the challenge is to implement these widely within existing systems (which may be slow to change, due to complex structures and funding systems) in a way that is theoretically informed and addresses policy concerns.

The Contributors

Professor June Andrews is the Director of the Dementia Services Development Centre at the University of Stirling, which improves services nationally and internationally for people with dementia and their carers through organisational change, information provision, research and training. A psychiatric and general trained nurse, she was formerly the director of the Centre for Change and Innovation, an NHS Board Director of Nursing, and the Secretary of the Royal College of Nursing in Scotland. In 2011 she was awarded the Robert Tiffany award for internationalization, and the British American Project Founders award for public service.

Sandrine Andrieu MD, PhD is a Professor of Epidemiology and Public Health at Toulouse University. She studied epidemiology and obtained her PhD in Aging and Public Health in 2002. She runs the INSERM-Toulouse University UMR1027 research unit and the 'Aging and Alzheimer Disease' research team. She has published over 120 international papers and book chapters in the field of aging. She is involved in large intervention studies for neuro-degenerative disease (PLASA, GuidAge, MAPT) and large cohorts of Alzheimer disease patients (ICTUS, REAL.fr). As a member of the Toulouse Gerontopole, she coordinates the French Observatory of Research on Alzheimer's Disease.

Sube Banerjee is Professor of Mental Health and Ageing at the Institute of Psychiatry, King's College London, directing its Centre for Innovation and Evaluation in Mental Health. Clinically, he developed and directs the Croydon Memory Service, a team for early diagnosis and treatment of dementia. He was the Department of Health for England's senior professional advisor on dementia and led the development of its National Dementia Strategy. An active researcher with more than 100 peer reviewed publications including work on: quality of life in dementia; psychosocial research; RCTs and the interface between policy, research and practice.

Claudine Berr, Medical Epidemiologist and Research Director at INSERM, is head of the 'Age-related cognitive disorders' team in the INSERM U1061 research unit in Montpellier. She has been the scientific coordinator of the Montpellier center of the 'Three-City study' since 2005. She has been working on the epidemiology of neurodegenerative diseases since 1990, mainly on the factors associated with the occurrence of cognitive impairment in the elderly and Alzheimer's disease, and combines clinical and epidemiological approaches to better understand the natural history of Alzheimer's disease in the general population.

Nicola Coley is an epidemiology and public health post-doc in INSERM-Toulouse University research unit UMR1027. She obtained her PhD in epidemiology in 2010, and her thesis was entitled 'Methodological Aspects of Clinical Trials for the Prevention and Treatment of Alzheimer's Disease'. She is involved in large Alzheimer's prevention trials (GuidAge, MAPT), and the ACCEPT study, studying the determinants of participation in prevention trials. She is a member of the French National Alzheimer Methodologies Group, providing methodological advice for clinical research projects on Alzheimer's disease, and is in charge of the French Observatory of Research on Alzheimer's Disease's clinical trials registry.

Loren deVries is Nurse Practitioner (Dementia Care) at The Garrawarra Centre, NSW Health, Australia, a specialist dementia care nursing home facility for individuals experiencing psychological and behavioural symptoms of dementia. Key achievements include a reduction in psychoactive medication use and increased effectiveness of pain management. Loren also held positions as an Area Clinical Nurse Consultant (Delirium and Dementia) across acute care services and a Research Associate leading a project in an aged care organization. Loren was awarded her Master's degrees in 2009 and 2011 (Nurse Practitioner from the University of Newcastle and Gerontology and Rehabilitation Studies from the University of Wollongong).

Dr Amit Dias is an Epidemiologist and Geriatrician by training and is currently the Professor at the Department of Preventive and Social Medicine at Goa Medical College. Dr Dias is the founder secretary of the Dementia Society of Goa and the coordinator of the 10/66 dementia research group in India. He is also the coordinator of the Medical and Scientific Advisory Panel for the Alzheimer's and Related Disorders Society of India. He was one of the authors of the National Dementia Report that was presented to the Government of India. He has a number of publications to his credit in national and international peer reviewed journals. His research on interventions for families of people with dementia won the International FMA-ADI prize for being the best evidence based psychosocial research in 2010. He also serves on the Managing committee of Sangath – an NGO working on mental health research and services in Goa, India.

Scott Dudgeon is a health policy consultant with 30 years' leadership experience in health care. In his current capacity, he authored *Rising Tide: The Impact of Dementia on Canadian Society*, and has helped Ontario to develop its mental health strategy, and is working with the Mental Health Commission of Canada in developing an investment case for mental health. Scott's prior experience includes leading the Alzheimer Society of Canada, the Canadian Collaborative Mental Health Initiative, Toronto District Health Council and Humber Memorial Hospital. Scott lives in Toronto and is active in his community, with extensive hospital and foundation board experience.

Emily Gallagher graduated with an MBChB from the University of Edinburgh in June 2010 and is currently an FY2 doctor working in south-east Scotland. Once she has completed her foundation training she will be working to Australia for 12 months and applying for core medical training with a view to a career in geriatric medicine.

Marie-Jo Guisset Martinez, after studying philosophy and social work, is Programmes Manager in Fondation Médéric Alzheimer, France, building up innovative issues to promote, support and evaluate new initiatives dedicated to people with dementia, their caregivers and professionals all around the country. She belongs currently to a number of research and practice European networks in dementia care. Her last publication, 'Regaining Identity: New synergies for a different approach to Alzheimer's' (Paris 2011), is available in French and Spanish.

Anthea Innes PhD is Professor of Health and Social Care Research at Bournemouth University, UK. She previously worked at the University of Stirling, where she was responsible for the development of the first MSc in Dementia Studies to be delivered using online learning. She has published widely with particular research interests in rural dementia care, technology, and the experiences of people with dementia and their carers.

Chris Johnson PhD is a retired Professor of Gerontology and Sociology at the University of Louisiana at Monroe (ULM). He developed the only Master's program in Gerontology in Louisiana, expanding it to be one the first online Masters of Gerontology programs in the South. He has published extensively in dementia, thanatology, gerontology, and sociology. He successfully authored grants and secured private donations for several million dollars for ULM. He is also a licensed professional counselor and marriage and family therapist. As a recent visiting Professor in Scotland, he taught and presented papers at universities located in Stirling, St. Andrews and Edinburgh.

Roxanna Johnson MS, CTRS is a Gerontologist, certified Recreation Therapist, and a PhD student in Dementia Studies at the University of Stirling in Scotland. Currently she is the Executive Director of Aging Consultants Incorporated, a company that provides educational seminars, staff training, and program evaluations for senior health care services. She has published widely in various journals blending the current research literature and her work experiences in nursing homes and assisted living facilities. Her research interests include cross-national comparisons of dementia care workers in nursing homes; designing dementia-friendly environments and developing therapeutic activity programs that promote chemical- and restraint-free settings.

Fiona Kelly PhD is a Lecturer in Dementia Studies at the University of Stirling. She is also a practicing nurse in the care of people with dementia. Her interests, in which she bridges practice and academia, include palliative and end of life care of people with dementia, design for people with dementia and communication and expressions of selfhood.

Louise McCabe PhD is a Lecturer in Dementia Studies at the University of Stirling. Her research interests focus on people with dementia and associated policy and practice issues. To date published work has included research on social policy and services for people with dementia in the UK and India; policy and service issues for people with alcohol related dementia; and frontline health and social care staff. Her current research grants bring together an interest in how lifestyle choices around health, exercise and alcohol use can influence the experiences of people with dementia. She also teaches on undergraduate and postgraduate dementia studies courses at the University of Stirling.

Emma Reynish completed her clinical training in geriatric medicine and internal medicine between posts in Britain (Edinburgh) and France (Toulouse). She coordinated the European Alzheimer's Disease Consortium and was involved in a number of multicentre European research projects on Alzheimer's disease. She returned to the UK in 2008 to work as a consultant geriatrician and is now involved in significant clinical quality improvement work. Her clinical activity involves acute geriatrics, community hospital work and a large medical memory clinic along with on call for acute medicine. Ongoing research includes work on dementia prevalence and outcomes.

Charles Scerri PhD is a Senior Lecturer in Neuropathology and Neuropharmacology at the Faculty of Medicine and Surgery, University of Malta. His research interests focus on the behavioural, biochemical, pharmacological and social aspects of Alzheimer's disease and associated dementias. He is a board member of Alzheimer Europe and acted as Chairperson of the Malta Dementia Strategy Working Group within the Ministry of Health. Recently he authored the document 'Inspiring New Frontiers – Recommendations for a Dementia Strategy in the Maltese Islands'.

Paulina Szymczynska has a background in psychology and management. She currently works as a Research Officer at Rethink Mental Illness and as a Teaching Assistant on undergraduate dementia studies modules at the University of Stirling. She has been involved in research with academic, public and voluntary institutions. She is particularly interested in the ways in which evidence is translated into mental health services practice and the impact of care and support on different stakeholder groups.

Laura Telford MBChB graduated from the University of Aberdeen in June 2010. She is currently working as an FY2 in the south-east Deanery in Scotland and intends to work in Australia from August 2012, before embarking on a career in General Practice.

Victoria Traynor is an Associate Professor in the School of Nursing, Midwifery and Indigenous Health, University of Wollongong, Australia. She is an Associate Director of the NSW and ACT Dementia Training Study Centre and coordinates Masters of Science degrees (Dementia Care and Geronotology and Rehabilitation Studies). Recent research projects include the development of 'Delirium Care Pathways' for the Australian Government and a model of person-centred care for Aboriginal and Torres Strait Islander communities. Previous positions were held with the University of Nottingham, RCN Institute and Oxford Brookes University. Victoria was awarded her PhD in 2001 from the University of Edinburgh.

Subject Index

Author Index